A Functional Medicine Monograph

DEPRESSION:
Advancing the Treatment Paradigm

Robert Hedaya, MD
Sheila Quinn

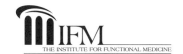

THE INSTITUTE FOR FUNCTIONAL MEDICINE

A Nonprofit Educational Organization
www.functionalmedicine.org

Depression: Advancing the Treatment Paradigm
Bob Hedaya, MD, and Sheila Quinn

Copyright ©2008, The Institute for Functional Medicine
4411 Pt. Fosdick Dr NW, Ste 305
P.O. Box 1697
Gig Harbor, WA 98335
800-228-0622
www.functionalmedicine.org

Disclaimer

This publication is intended only for use as an educational tool to broaden the knowledge and perspective of health practitioners. Nothing herein is intended to substitute for an individualized, thoughtful decision process by patients and providers. Clinically related material is not presented as a prescription for treatment, but rather as an indicator of the kind of information clinicians may want to consider in making treatment decisions for their patients. Neither the publisher, the authors, the editors, nor the reviewer assume any liability for any injury and/or damage to persons or property arising from the information to be found in this publication.

Project Team
Allison Templet, Project Manager, Editor, and Contributing Writer
Jay Lombard, DO, Technical Reviewer
Mary Smith, Cover Design
D. Kari Luraas, Interior Design and Layout
Lynn Siefken, Illustrator

ISBN-10: 0-9773713-4-4
ISBN-13: 978-0-9773713-4-1

Contents

Continuing Medical Education General Information v

Preface ix

Section I   **Introduction and Background** 1

Chapter 1   **History and Prevailing Views** 3

Historical Development of the Concept of Depression 3
Current Prevailing Views 14
Integrative Summary 16
References 17

Chapter 2   **The Cultural Context of Depression** 19

Depression in Western Culture 19
Depression in Other Cultures 20
Summary 21
References 21

Chapter 3   **Epidemiology and Public Health Impact** 23

The Epidemiology of Depression 23
Public Health Impact of Depression 25
References 36

Section II   **State of the Science in Assessment and Treatment** 41

Chapter 4   **Drug Treatments for Depression** 43

Drug Classes and Mechanisms: A Brief Review 43
Antidepressant Outcomes and Limitations of the Evidence 50
Strategies for Enhancing Antidepressant Effectiveness 51
References 52

Contents

Chapter 5   **Psychotherapy and Other Conventional Treatments**..55

    Psychotherapy.. 55
    Other Treatments for Depression... 56
    New Directions.. 58
    References... 58

Chapter 6   **Mechanisms and Interconnections within the Functional Medicine Matrix Model** 61

    Hormone and Neurotransmitter Regulation 61
    Immune Surveillance 67
    Inflammatory Process... 68
    Digestion, Absorption, and Barrier Integrity 69
    Detoxification and Biotransformation 70
    Oxidative/Reductive Homeodynamics 71
    Structural Integrity... 72
    Psychological and Spiritual Equilibrium 73
    Nutritional Status... 73
    References... 78

Section III   **Clinical Applications** 85

Chapter 7   **Clinical Discussion: Experiences in Assessment and Treatment** 87

    Structuring the Clinical Management of Depression: A Systems Approach 88
    The Interview: Critical Steps in Eliciting the Depressed Patient's Story 89
    Using the Functional Medicine Matrix Model 94
    A — Assessment Strategies 95
    B — Clinical Interventions 99
    C — Practical Implications and Considerations... 110
    References... 112

Chapter 8   **Clinical Cases** 115

    Case History — Carl 115
    Case History — Benjamin 116
    Case History — Heather 118
    Case History — Mark 121
    Case History—Tamika 123
    References... 124

Appendix   **Medical Symptoms Questionnaire** 125

About the Authors 129

Continuing Medical Education General Information

Accreditation Statement

The Institute for Functional Medicine (IFM) is accredited by the Accreditation Council for Continuing Medical Education (ACCME) to provide continuing medical education (CME) for physicians.

Commercial Support

This CME activity is supported by educational grants from Doctor's Data Inc., Genova Diagnostics, InnoVision Health Media Inc., Metagenics, Inc., Metametrix Clinical Laboratory, Nordic Naturals, Inc., SpectraCell Laboratories, Inc., Thorne Research, Inc., TID*health*, Vital Nutrients, Vitamin Research Products, and Xymogen.

Continuing Education Credit Designations

For MDs and DOs, IFM designates this educational activity for a maximum of 6 *AMA PRA Category 1 credit(s)™*. Physicians should only claim credit commensurate with the extent of their participation in the activity.

Release date: May 22, 2008
Expiration date: May 22, 2011
Medium: Monograph

Method of Participation

To obtain CME credit for your participation in this activity:

1. Please read this monograph.
2. Complete the online evaluation, which will be sent to you via e-mail after purchase of the monograph; if you have any questions about accessing or completing the evaluation, contact IFM Client Services by e-mailing client_services@fxmed.com or calling 800-228-0622.

Statement of Need

Gap analyses and needs assessments conducted by IFM demonstrate an urgency for education and new approaches to the treatment of depression. The research reveals a global epidemic of depression, with more than half of depressed patients with only partial or no recovery using standard medical therapies. Depression is a complex, multifactorial condition that is comorbid with many chronic diseases, demanding a new approach that identifies and addresses the common underlying metabolic dysregulations. This monograph bridges the gap between current and best practice by presenting a comprehensive, systems-oriented approach to solving the problem of depression.

Learning Objectives

- Improve chronic disease outcomes by recognizing the common metabolic dysfunctions that underlie both depression and its comorbid conditions.
- Evaluate the effectiveness of conventional treatments for depression, including drugs and psychotherapy, and utilize such treatments when appropriate.
- Identify and remediate the dysregulated metabolic pathways and processes that can influence neuronal function and mood, including hormonal imbalance, oxidative stress, digestion, inflammation, infection, and detoxification.
- Determine which patients with depression will benefit from diet, nutritional, hormonal, and pharmacological therapies
- Utilize history taking, interviewing, and laboratory/genomic testing techniques, in the evaluation of patients presenting with depression.
- Effectively distinguish between atypical and melancholic depression in order to optimize care.

Purpose Statement

The purpose of this monograph is to provide an expanded assessment and treatment model of depression. The scientific rationale for this comprehensive approach will be presented, and functional medicine interventions will be described from both the theoretical and practical perspectives.

Who Should Participate?

Any physician who cares for patients with chronic depression, including primary care and specialist physicians.

Objectivity and Independence

It is the policy of IFM that all CME activities sponsored by IFM shall provide independent, balanced, objective, and scientifically rigorous presentations that are free of commercial bias. In accordance with ACCME Essential Areas and policies, IFM is totally responsible for all decisions on key components of activity development, including the development of activity goals and objectives, promotional material, content, faculty selection and approval, activity evaluation, and maintenance of physicians' credits.

Policy on Disclosure

As a sponsor accredited by ACCME, it is the policy of IFM to require all planners, authors, and editors to disclose (1) the existence of any relevant financial relationships with the supporters of this activity or manufacturer(s) of any commercial product(s) or services(s) that are discussed in their presentation, and (2) references in their presentations to unlabeled or unapproved use of drugs or devices. Disclosures are provided below.

Author Disclosure Statements

Bob Hedaya, MD, has indicated he has no financial relationships with any relevant commercial supporter or with the manufacturer of any commercial product or provider of any commercial service relevant to this activity

Sheila Quinn has indicated she has no financial relationships with any relevant commercial supporter or with the manufacturer of any commercial product or provider of any commercial service relevant to this activity.

Content Planner Disclosure Statements

David Jones, MD, is President and Director of Medical Education of the Institute for Functional Medicine.

Dan Lukaczer, ND, is Associate Director of Medical Education of the Institute for Functional Medicine.

Allison Templet is project editor and coordinator at the Institute for Functional Medicine.

Preface

Several years ago, The Institute for Functional Medicine (IFM) conducted a detailed needs assessment of clinicians to help in our program planning process. Among the top three needs uncovered was a better approach to the treatment of depression. The urgency and volume of the responses generated IFM's commitment to the monograph you are about to read—a breakthrough exploration of functional medicine applications to assessing and treating depression.

The research quickly lays bare the reasons that practitioners are feeling such urgency, even desperation, about the need for better tools to treat depression. Not only is there an epidemic of depression globally, but the current conventional paradigm leaves more than half of depressed patients with only partial or no recovery. Despite the very significant relief experienced by many patients treated with drugs and psychotherapy, far too many others are not adequately helped by those treatments. Undoubtedly, that fact weighs heavily in the thoughts of clinicians everywhere.

We are extremely—perhaps uniquely—fortunate to have secured for our primary author of this monograph the expertise and dedication of a psychiatrist who came to the functional medicine paradigm many years ago and who has tested and refined his use of functional medicine. His expertise is broad, deep, and solidly rooted in both clinical practice and the evolving science. Robert Hedaya, MD, author, professor of psychiatry at Georgetown University, and founder of the National Center for Whole Psychiatry in Chevy Chase, Maryland, has made a personal commitment to sharing his knowledge and skills with colleagues around the world. This monograph, in preparation for more than a year, deeply reflects his views and his clinical practice, and we honor and appreciate him for his generosity and dedication in making this information available.

Descriptions and correlates of what we now call depressive disorders are present in much of recorded history. There is an amazing persistence of concepts and symptoms, and even of certain hypotheses about causes. This monograph reflects knowledge and judgment at a point in time and from a specific perspective, but assuredly it is not the final answer. Our understanding continues to evolve. What we bring to the table today, for clinicians and their patients, is a comprehensive, systems-oriented approach to thought and practice in solving the problem of depression—a way to think critically about the myriad factors involved in etiology, treatment, and prevention, including lifestyle (diet, stress, exercise, spiritual practices), genetic vulnerabilities (family history, polymorphisms), and environment (workplace influences, toxic exposures in air, water, and food, neighborhood safety, isolation). We use functional medicine concepts and constructs to help organize both the information and the critical thinking process.

Ultimately, a picture emerges that strongly validates depression as a complex, multifactorial condition that is comorbid with many chronic diseases and that shares many underlying metabolic dysregulations with those conditions. Like the depression itself, these underlying dysregulations often go unrecognized. Even when diagnosed, depression is too frequently not treated to full recovery. Depression is very likely a causal—and certainly a contributing—factor in a number of very serious (and costly) conditions. It is fueled by a variety of underlying imbalances in physiology and biochemistry that we, as clinicians, must become better at detecting, assessing, and treating. Realistically, when managing depression (or, indeed, any chronic disease), we must address not only the primary condition, but all the significant comorbidities and underlying dysfunctions as well, if we hope to bring our patients to full and lasting recovery. This is a significant challenge for clinicians in today's healthcare environment, but it's difficult to overstate the huge impact of this interconnected web: depression now afflicts more than 120 million people worldwide! It is our deepest hope that presenting the functional medicine approach to identification, assessment, and treatment of depression will bring relief and recovery to many who have thus far sought it in vain.

We acknowledge the greater difficulty of assessing and treating such a varied assortment of triggers and mediators of depression—surely, it is simpler in this era of managed care to write a prescription or recommend psychotherapy. While those approaches are not to be discarded, clinicians from all disciplines recognize that they are not enough for far too many people. Thus, we are called to learn (and teach) this new approach, just as we were called to medicine in the first place. It is our responsibility to ensure that the best of our knowledge and skill is available to our patients. This monograph is dedicated to that outcome.

The difficulty in integrating such a mass of diverse information and conveying it in an intelligible and accessible manner required a rare skill. We are deeply indebted to coauthor Sheila Quinn for nothing less than a supremely masterful contribution. Many thanks to the rest of the team that supported Dr. Hedaya in producing this monograph: Dan Lukaczer, ND, IFM associate director of medical education; Allison Templet, project manager, editor, and contributing writer; and Jay Lombard, DO, technical reviewer. They have done an outstanding job.

As always, let us know your thoughts about this publication; your feedback will strengthen our understanding of the usefulness and accuracy of the information and will help all of us to continue advancing the paradigm.

David S. Jones, MD
President and Director of Medical Education
The Institute for Functional Medicine

Section I

Introduction and Background

While identification and management of depressive mood disorders has advanced considerably in the past 50 years with the advent of various assessment tools, medications, and other therapies, the need for improved assessment and treatment of depression as a primary condition, as a comorbid condition, and as a critical factor in the effort to improve outcomes in the larger arena of chronic disease is of paramount importance.

Our goal in this section of the monograph is to establish the urgent need for an expanded assessment and treatment model of depression.[i] Chapter 1 will provide a historical context for the monograph, tracing the development of some core concepts through changes in language, etiology, and treatment. It's notable that, despite myriad variations and scientific developments, depression is still an extremely challenging condition to identify and treat successfully. Chapter 2 will offer some thoughts on cultural issues that play a role in the prevalence and incidence of depression, and Chapter 3 will establish the scope and nature of the problem on a population level, in addition to analyzing the public health impact of a disease that is extremely widespread and that has myriad profound connections to other chronic diseases. In subsequent chapters (4, 5, and 6), we will develop the scientific rationale for integrating a functional medicine approach into a comprehensive strategy for treating depression. And in the final chapters (7 and 8), we will present functional medicine interventions from both theoretical and practical perspectives (including case studies).

---

[i] It's important to note that this monograph addresses only unipolar depression. While treatment concepts may be relevant to manic depression or mania alone, that is not our focus.

Chapter 1

History and Prevailing Views

Historical Development of the Concept of Depression

Although the concept of depression as a disease emerged relatively late in history, melancholic moods have been noted by medical writers (and in Western literature) for at least 5000 years.[ii] It is a topic whose complexity and tenacity have driven the evolution of diverse theories for millennia. While the concepts, language, and definitions have all undergone myriad shifts throughout this long period, it is important to note that several ideas have remained strikingly consistent in the history of melancholia (the older term) and depression (the modern term):

- **Mood and affect** — Alterations of both subjective emotional experience (mood) and objective manifestations of altered emotion (affect) are often described as sadness; alterations in these parameters to an intensity and duration beyond that which is generally understandable from the person's life circumstances become recognizable symptoms of the disturbance.
- **Genetics** — What today might be called genetic predisposition has been acknowledged using terms such as *melancholy by nature* or *congenital temperament*.
- **Individuality** — Such illnesses take many different guises (i.e., manifestations vary a great deal among different patients) and have multifactorial, variable, and often unknown causes, including hormonal shifts.
- **Multifactorial causation** — Diet, environment (including family and occupation), upbringing, and lifestyle influence both the causation and course of the condition.
- **Spirituality** — Connections between the spiritual/religious domains and melancholia have long been recognized.

In the common mind and language, no real distinction was made between disease and temperament in relation to melancholia until the modern era, nor were distinctions made between melancholia/depression and schizophrenia, so any historical discussion using modern terminology is bound to contain anachronistic elements.[1] Bearing in mind that terminology, culture, and treatment have varied widely over the millennia, there is sufficient value in a brief historical review of what is today a widely recognized, pervasive, and debilitating disease to override the valid concerns about what is lost when history is so compressed.

We will not define in this brief review all the terms used throughout history or what they might have meant within the cultures and languages of their times. It is important to note, however, that the boundary between the affective disorders and the schizophrenic disorders has been debated since the early 1900s by 2 schools of thought:

[ii] Details provided here on the history of depression through 1985 owe a great debt to Stanley W. Jackson's 1986 book *Melancholia and Depression: From Hippocratic Times to Modern Times*, which is well referenced and frequently cited by more recent authors examining the history of depression. Unless otherwise referenced, most of this chapter was developed by extracting, distilling, and paraphrasing extensive information from Jackson's work on key trends and influential figures; any errors that have surfaced in this process are those of the authors and should not be attributed to Jackson.

Job: A Biblical "Case"

The book of Job is thought by some scholars to be the oldest book in the Bible. The literary form of Job is similar to documents that date to the first part of the 2nd millennium BCE. It is remarkable that this ancient text should provide insight into the psycho-social-spiritual subject that we have now collapsed into the single word depression. The survival of this document for over 4000 years is a testament to the enduring and widespread nature of the depressive experience, as well as its relevance to the deeper question with which all sentient beings struggle at one time or another: What is the meaning of life? While it is difficult for the modern mind to conceive of illness as having any value, a depth psychological perspective does view illness as the psyche's attempt to get the individual to pay attention to matters of soul. The body and mind are the courts of last resort for the psyche. In this sense, if illness is attended to as meaningful and as a messenger, then the individual is called to do the work of soul tending. It is this nonmaterial level of existence to which the book of Job directs us.

In biblical times, the causal attribution of depression was clearly spiritual: "Satan went out from the presence of the LORD and afflicted Job with painful sores from the soles of his feet to the top of his head."* Job, a very wealthy, prosperous, and pious man, was suddenly faced with the loss of all his possessions, as well as the death of all of his sons and daughters. What follows are quotations from the book of Job that illustrate the unchanging nature of the core experience of depression through the millennia.

1. **Passive suicidal ideation** — "Why did I not perish at birth, and die as I came from the womb? I despise my life; I would not live forever."

2. **Anxiety/obsessiveness** — "I have no peace, no quietness; I have no rest, but only turmoil. When I think about this, I am terrified; trembling seizes my body."

3. **Hopelessness** — "What strength do I have, that I should still hope? What prospects, that I should be patient?"

4. **Insomnia** — "When I lie down I think, 'How long before I get up?' The night drags on, and I toss till dawn."

5. **Infection/inflammation/malnutrition, poor self-care** — "My body is clothed with worms and scabs, my skin is broken and festering. My breath is offensive to my wife."

6. **Social withdrawal, loss of meaning** — "Let me alone; my days have no meaning."

7. **Anhedonia** — "My days are swifter than a runner; they fly away without a glimpse of joy."

8. **Social ostracism** — "I am loathsome to my own brothers. Even the little boys scorn me; when I appear, they ridicule me. All my intimate friends detest me; those I love have turned against me."

9. **Failure of treatment** — "…you are worthless physicians, all of you! …Your maxims are proverbs of ashes; your defenses are defenses of clay…. I have heard many things like these; miserable comforters are you all! Will your long-winded speeches never end? What ails you that you keep on arguing? … So how can you console me with your nonsense? Nothing is left of your answers but falsehood!"

10. **Reduced appetite, weight loss** — "I am nothing but skin and bones."

* All quotations from the book of Job, New International Version, at http://www.biblegateway.com/passage/?search=Job%201:1-2:10&version=31

Kraepelinian[2] and Bleulerian.[3] In general, Europeans have favored an approach that diagnosed individuals as schizophrenic if they were on the boundary (i.e., the person seemed depressed but had hallucinations or delusions), while American psychiatry included many schizophrenics under the diagnosis of depression, even if there were psychotic features. This gap has narrowed, as American psychiatry has moved in the direction of the Europeans, and there is now a schizoaffective diagnostic category in American nosology.

Hippocratic Times

Hippocratic writings in the 5th and 4th centuries BCE suggest that a disease called melancholia had already been identified by the ancient physicians. They believed that it was caused by an imbalance in the 4 humors (blood, yellow bile, black bile, and phlegm), specifically by an excess of black bile (associated with dryness and coolness). Its primary characteristics were startlingly similar to symptoms associated with certain depressive disorders today—despondency, sleeplessness, irritability, restlessness, aversion to food. Even the concept of chronicity had already surfaced ("fear or depression that is prolonged means melancholia"[4]). Aristotle may have been the first to hypothesize that depression was frequently associated with artistic and intellectual gifts (perhaps an indication of the manic, creative aspects of the disorder in some individuals), and that theme has recurred periodically through the centuries.

By the time of Galen (2nd and 3rd centuries CE), a constellation of melancholic diseases was clearly noted, of which melancholia was one. Between Hippocrates and Galen, the humoral theory had undergone many minor variations—and was to undergo many more—but it lasted with remarkable consistency for over 2000 years, only coming under serious challenge in the 18th century and finally dying out in the 19th. Galen identified a number of causes for the excess of black bile, including various foods and occupations, sleeplessness and anxiety, seasons, stages of life (perhaps thereby hinting at the hormonal impact of pregnancy, birth, and menopause), and even geography ("cold and dry modes of life, regions, constitutions"[4]). Treatments included dietary recommendations, baths (hydrotherapy), exercise, massage, and stimulation of blood flow, which included reestablishing menstruation (early recognition of hormonal factors) and even encouraging hemorrhoidal flow. Bloodletting as a treatment emanated from various aspects of the humoral theory of causation and did not die out until that theory was finally abandoned.

Medieval Times

Greek medicine was disseminated throughout the world via translations and compilations of the writings of Galen and Hippocrates, although the development of Byzantine medicine (centered in Alexandria) diverged substantially during the early Middle Ages from the ideas that evolved in the primarily Christian traditions of Western and Northern Europe, where the influence of religion was evident in the notion that mental illnesses were punishments by God of sinful behavior (see *Job: A Biblical "Case"*). The concentration of literacy in the monasteries, where the translating, compiling, and interpreting of the ancient texts became deeply steeped in prevailing religious thought, was a major factor in this divergence. During the Islamic Middle Ages, however, concepts based upon the Greek writings, which were focused more on medicine and culture than on religion, continued to develop. In the 13th century, Latin translations of many of the Arabic and Greek texts were finally brought fairly widely to the (literate) Western world, and the divergent traditions began to converge again.

Maimonides (1135–1204 CE), a Jewish rabbi, physician, and philosopher in Spain, Morocco, and Egypt during the Middle Ages, was the most famous physician in the medieval world. He wrote 10 major treatises on medicine. Perhaps as a result of experiencing a major depression coincident with the death of his father and younger brother in the same year, he "put the treatment of mental illness on an equal footing as that of physical illness, insisting, for example, that the physician provide immediate psychiatric care following a suicide attempt."[5] He wrote of the importance of the body-mind connection and vividly described the mourning that is associated with loss, as well as the inability to anticipate pleasure or happiness in the future.[6] His writings were known to every important medical tradition in the Judeo-Christian-Arabic world of his time and for centuries thereafter.

Within the Christian church, the condition of acedia—characterized by apathy, sadness, restlessness, and exhaustion—was deemed a cardinal sin, which those who lived within the monastic traditions had particularly to guard against. The belief in confession and penance as medicine for the soul took hold, and the condition gradually became connected to the concept of spiritual idleness or neglect, for which busyness was thought to be the antidote. This would be but an interesting sidelight except that, in the minds of many, acedia (the sin) was often confused with melancholia (the disease), and therefore both conditions were believed to have moral and religious causation and cure (a belief not entirely unknown even today). Both Petrarch and Chaucer, for example, portrayed acedia in terms very similar to those used to describe melancholia: grief, sorrow, dejection (Petrarch); and heaviness, sorrow, despair, moodiness, anger, and neglect of duty (Chaucer). This construct did not include delusions, but it was known that the condition could advance to the point of suicide. Although the medical frame of reference for melancholia was less concerned with sin and duty and more interested in physiology, some aspects of the concept of acedia were nonetheless absorbed into the definitions of melancholia and were perpetuated in medical thinking until the modern era (although lessening in importance from the Renaissance forward).

The Renaissance

Baroque and Renaissance art both contain famous examples of the melancholic temperament,[7] demonstrating its emergence into the popular culture. Until the 16th century, medicine was basically Galenic, an orientation that gave way only slowly under the weight of new ideas about science and medicine. The 15th and 16th centuries were noted for their contributions to anatomy (Vesalius) and physiology (Harvey) and the beginnings of medical chemistry and surgery (Park). Bedside teaching of medical skills began in this period, and diagnostic categories begin to emerge with better definition and consistency. There were at least as many views of melancholia at that time, however, as there are of depression today.

By the time of the Renaissance, a differentiation between mania and depression had been noted, although those labels would converge and diverge many times before the end of the 20th century. Paracelsus (1493–1541) identified 4 types of insanity, of which melancholia was one. He disagreed with the clergy's view of mental disorders as supernatural in origin, thus helping to weaken the religious influence on concepts of mental illness. A treatise by Andre Du Laurens, *Melancholike Diseases*, written in the late 16th century, stood as the primary Renaissance review of medical thought since Galen. Du Laurens was still entrenched in the humoral theory of causation (with some variations), and he described 3 categories of mental illness (frensie, madness, and melancholia),[4] which we might very loosely compare to mania, schizophrenia, and depression today. In Du Laurens, fear and sadness were again reported as major characteristics of melancholia, as well as other somatic symptoms (gastrointestinal disturbances, fatigue, various aches and pains); the connection to the "gifted" individual was also noted, describing a link between mood disorders, creativity, and exuberance. Treatments involved sleep, exercise, diet, air, and company (afflicted individuals were not to be left alone), as well as diminutives (purging and bloodletting), alteratives (to moisten and warm, such as baths, broths, and syrups), and *comfortatives* (opiates and other soothing substances)—all categories of treatment that continued to be recommended for several more centuries and modern versions of which can still be found today.

René Descartes (1596–1650) was a highly influential French philosopher, mathematician, scientist, and writer. Often called the founder of modern philosophy, much of subsequent Western philosophy is a reaction to his writings. Descartes believed that the body works like a machine and that it follows the laws of physics. The mind, however, was described as a nonmaterial entity that does not follow the laws of physics. Separating the mind and body into distinct entities obeying different laws created what is known as *Cartesian dualism*, a dichotomy that set the agenda for philosophical discussions of the mind-body problem for many years after Descartes's death. In a very real sense, this Cartesian duality continues to pervade modern views about causality and approaches to depression, although more integrative thinking today encompasses both/and (body and mind), rather than either/or.

The Anatomy of Melancholy by Robert Burton,[8] published in 1621, described melancholy as a disease, a humor, and a temperament, representing the 3 major views of the complex condition in this time and culture. Although causation was still thought to be humoral at this point, the involvement of the brain was more fully described. The 3 types of melancholia were thought to be: (1) a primary condition of the brain, (2) a generalized condition in which brain involvement was secondary, and (3) primary involvement of hypochondriacal regions with secondary involvement of the brain (this latter condition being associated with somatic symptoms, particularly flatulence).

The Age of Enlightenment

Thus, by the 17th century, "melancholia had been an established clinical syndrome… for approximately two thousand years,"[4] with little fundamental alteration in concepts of causation or treatment. The 17th century initiated a major break with medieval thought and philosophy, as well as with medicine. It is often called the Age of Reason and is considered to precede the Age of Enlightenment or to actually be the earlier part of the Enlightenment, which was primarily concentrated in the 18th century.

Barbara Ehrenreich recently wrote: "There is reason to think that something like an epidemic of depression… began around 1600," starting in England and eventually striking most of Europe.[9] "The disease attacked young and old, plunging them into months or years of morbid lethargy and relentless terrors, and seemed… to single out men of accomplishment and genius," such as John Bunyan, Oliver Cromwell, Thomas Gray, John Donne, and Samuel Johnson (again making an association with the creative manic aspects of the disorder). Ehrenreich raised intriguing questions about the extent to which the rise in melancholia paralleled the evolution of society from one in which each person's role and identity were fixed and unchangeable into one that allowed for upward mobility and personal growth; this new society created a sense of personal autonomy, but perhaps also a growing sense of isolation and separation from the larger community, as well as the anxiety and self-judgment that often accompany personal responsibility for behavior and success. Ehrenreich pointed out that the communal pleasures of singing and dancing that accompanied medieval festivals declined as urbanization arose and Church repression of joyful expression prevailed, unfortunately eliminating an effective antidote to melancholia just when it was most needed. If there is any truth in these hypotheses, then it would not be surprising that the epidemic of depression has only intensified as industrialization, urbanization, and alienation have blanketed so much of modern human culture, and pleasures have increasingly become solitary and cerebral, rather than communal and physical.

Toward the end of the 17th century, ideas about pathogenesis began to take shape, together with an emerging knowledge of body chemistry and biomechanics. By the mid-1700s, however, mechanistic theories about melancholia (such as circulatory obstruction or retardation) were already being debunked, and electricity had emerged as a medical/physiological explanation. The vitalistic tradition was coming to the fore in medicine, and scientific experimentation was becoming common. Newtonian etherial notions (a "subtle spirit" pervades bodies and creates attractions and repulsions between cells, affecting nerves, muscles and the brain) heralded the shift of emphasis to the brain and nervous system that displaced the hydraulic/mechanical theories about melancholia centered on the heart and vascular system (although Freudian theory of the early 1900s drew extensively on this hydraulic mechanistic model in descriptions of the id, the ego, and the superego). And in drama, women's vulnerability to melancholia as a result of the hormonal changes of pregnancy (or disappointments in love) also presaged the feminization of depression.[1]

A sharper distinction between madness/insanity (psychosis) and melancholia (partial insanity, or neurosis) emerged in the medical literature, and the use of the word depression to indicate both mood and disease was seen for the first time. Samuel Johnson, a sufferer through much of his life, wrote of *depression of spirits* and *depression of mind*,[1] although he did not offer any definitions for those terms in his famous *Dictionary of the English Language*.[10]

Entering the Modern Era

Straddling the 18th and 19th centuries, Philippe Pinel was a key figure in the simplification of a schema for mental illness. He described a 4-part construct, involving mania, melancholia, dementia, and idiotism. He reaffirmed melancholia as *partial insanity* (a term that had been much used in earlier times) and, although not the first to mention it, he clearly identified bipolarity (manic depression) as a form of melancholia. He retreated from any theories about causation, taking instead a phenomenological approach in which he considered individual outcomes as resulting from external effects on unique premorbid dispositions (foreshadowing the concept of genomics and the mechanisms of antecedents and triggers of illness). He noted that no organic lesions were typically found on autopsy of afflicted patients, and he thought that moral causes (e.g., "ungovernable or disappointed ambition, religious fanaticism, profound chagrin, and unfortunate love"[4]) predominated. He advocated *moral treatment*, characterized primarily as efforts to give the patient's thought patterns a new direction (foreshadowing cognitive therapy) by whatever means necessary, including clean and healthy surroundings, productive work (e.g., occupational therapy), and incentives for good behavior.[iii] Two significant contributions of the moral treatment movement were establishing a rationale for non-somatic treatment (e.g., psychological therapy) and viewing the patient as having an ability to participate actively in therapy—*a psychology of the autonomous mind*.[11]

Over the course of the 19th century, many new ideas about the causes, nature, and treatment of melancholia and depression arose. From Benjamin Rush (the father of American psychiatry) and his ideas about pathogenesis in fevers, to Jean-Étienne Esquirol who firmly disavowed the humoral theory and identified multiple causes (e.g., seasons, climates, aging, idleness, vocations, hereditary predispositions, domestic troubles, disappointment in love or finance), to Wilhelm Griesinger who described all forms of mental illness as stages within a single disease that stemmed from changes in the brain (the seeds of biological psychiatry) and were influenced by hereditary predisposition and upbringing, we begin to approach the modern era. In John Tuke and Daniel Bucknill's *Manual of Psychological Medicine*, published in 1858, the symptoms associated with a detailed classification system for mental illnesses are similar to current times; the essential predisposition is hereditary and precipitating causes are "moral" (with the meaning described above for moral causes and treatments). Tuke and Bucknill emphasized the importance of understanding cerebral pathology, including inflammation (foreshadowing the functional medicine approach), and recommended both moral treatment and dietary and lifestyle interventions, including cold baths, exercise, and fresh air; opiates for acute melancholia were also mentioned.

As psychiatry and psychology moved into the 20th century, Henry Maudsley was the first to identify "two great divisions—*Affective* and *Ideational*"[4] in the forms of insanity, and he used the presence or absence of delusions as the critical differentiating factor. He believed that affective disorders preceded ideational ones and stemmed from underlying cerebral dysfunction. Hereditary predisposition, upbringing, and life experiences were all thought to be influential, as they are considered today. Recommended treatments mirrored the Pinel, Tuke, and Bucknill approaches described above.

Richard von Krafft-Ebing, author of *Text-Book of Insanity* (perhaps the most influential clinical text in the last 2 decades of the 19th century), organized what he labeled as the *mental diseases of the adult brain* into functional psychoses (psychoneuroses and psychic degeneration) and organic psychoses. Among the 4 forms of psychoneuroses were melancholia and mania. He described melancholia as a painful emotional depression without sufficient observable cause that arises spontaneously and exists independently. Symptoms included insomnia, lack of energy, and loss of appetite and/or weight. Treatment was complete mental and physical rest, surveillance for protection (i.e., hospitalization), diet, warm baths, and opium for sleeplessness.

[iii] Moral treatment was brought to England in 1796 by the Tukes family, who established The Retreat, an asylum in which "moral treatment was cultivated as a non-medical therapy." [Laffey P. Psychiatric therapy in Georgian Britain. *Psychol Med*. 2003;33:1285-1297.]

The Early 20th Century (1900–1950)

Emil Kraepelin was a central figure in 20th century psychiatry, having evolved a new nosology that brought together all the various terms relating to melancholia under the heading *manic depressive insanity*, which he viewed as a single morbid process that had multiple expressions, including periodic and circular insanity, simple mania, melancholia, amentia, mood, and personal predisposition. He clarified that while the boundaries among these 6 conditions were fluid, none of them advanced into dementia. Treatment was essentially unchanged despite his observation that for melancholia of gradual development, prolonged duration, and gradual convalescence,[iv] one third recover and two thirds undergo further mental deterioration. Significantly, these are similar to response rates reported in recent research on conventional treatment. (See *Antidepressant Outcomes and Limitations of the Evidence* in Chapter 4.)

The distinction between endogenous (intangible, a result of predispositions—or, what's left when all exogenous causes are ruled out) and exogenous (caused by trauma, toxins, or any external and measurable etiology) depression was introduced by Paul Julius Möbius in 1893 and entered English language usage in the 1920s. Other polarities that were explored to characterize these distinctions were autonomous (sometimes called vegetative due to the prominence of impaired appetite and sleep)/reactive and primary/secondary. Endogenous/reactive eventually was replaced by the primary/secondary dichotomy, in an attempt to remove implications about etiology, but there were widely varying degrees of acceptance for all these terms across German, British, and American psychiatry, as reflected in early versions of the *Diagnostic and Statistical Manual of Mental Disorders* (DSM-I and -II). As Jackson so aptly stated, "Throughout the history of these various dichotomies, one finds recurrent evidence of the grand dualisms of nature-nurture and body-mind as underlying assumptions."[4]

Adolf Meyer, a dominant figure in American psychiatry between 1895 and 1940, conceived of psychiatric disorders as "maladaptive reaction patterns that depended on constitution and life experiences."[4] He argued for the elimination of the term melancholia from the lexicon in favor of depression and further revised the nosology to describe *affective reaction types* comprising manic depression, anxiety, series nervousness, and the simple depressions, which were excesses of normal depressions. In effect, he abandoned prognosis and etiology as nosological criteria in favor of a pragmatic approach. In treatment, he looked for points of modifiability as foci for intervention and change. He did not agree with hereditary dispositions and viewed the patient as collaborator in treatment, using psychotherapy that was kindly and humane, in addition to nutrition, sleep, baths, recreation, and socialization as important therapeutic tools.

David Henderson and R.D. Gillespie, publishers of a very influential British textbook series, continued to develop the classification of reaction types, including the Kraepelin concept of involutional melancholia. Although it is not necessary here to understand all the permutations of these concepts, it is worthwhile noting that, in 1944, Henderson and Gillespie changed the terminology for the first stage of depressive states to *simple depression* (thus eliminating the intermittent use of *retardation* to indicate the slowing of mental and physical processes often characteristic of depression) and added a section on electroconvulsive (ECT) or shock treatment.

Karl Abraham in 1911 provided the first extensive clinical-psychoanalytic data on severe depressive illnesses, in which he discerned a familial, constitutional factor, perceiving his patients as standing "helpless before the problems of life."[4] Soon thereafter, Sigmund Freud[12] published *Mourning and Melancholia* (1917). He used depression as both a descriptive term and a diagnostic one, but Freud's genius lay in the fact that (unlike virtually everyone else who preceded him) his view was that the etiology of depression was significantly psychological and unconscious: depression was related to unresolved ambivalent attachment to a person and subsequent loss. The patient had identified psychologically with, or taken in, another person (an introject), including the negative aspects, and then had become disdainful of those negative traits which now existed within the self. Because of the ambivalence toward the object, the patient is unable to mourn the loss in a normal way. The difference between normal grief (mourning) and

---

[iv]   Kraepelin and others have used the phrase *involutional melancholia* to identify this pattern. This term has gradually faded from use despite never having received a definitive analysis of whether it was a valid disease entity.

melancholia (depression) is the sense of emptiness: the individual who mourns feels that the world is empty, but the individual who is melancholic feels the emptiness and loss of self-esteem within. This inner emptiness was thought to be a result of the unconscious introjection of reproaches against the other. As a result of this conceptualization, many people credit Freud with the idea that depression is anger turned inward. In fact, however, that concept is a simplification of Freud's view. Clinicians who use the anger-turned-inward concept as a basis for motivating the depressed person to express anger sometimes find that this does not alleviate the depression but may increase the sense of guilt.

Freud originally believed that the primary causes of depression were biological; however, lacking adequate tools to explore this idea, he focused on the psychosexual etiology of depression, for which he identified 3 types: common, severe melancholia; neurasthenic melancholia; and anxious melancholia. He also distinguished between loss in the external world (observable) versus loss in ego, where cause is not apparent and therefore outcome seems puzzling. Both Freud and Abraham identified loss of love in infancy as a critical factor, and both were instrumental in the development of psychoanalysis as an independent therapeutic tool. However, research has failed to validate psychoanalysis as a useful treatment for depression (probably in part because of the difficulty of constructing a valid research model for studying the efficacy of psychoanalysis).[13]

Carl Jung, a junior contemporary of Freud, was initially mentored by Freud himself. However, in a sharp departure from Freud, Jung abandoned the mechanistic, left-brain, pathology-based model developed by Freud. He did not focus on specific symptoms or syndromes such as depression or hysteria, nor did he believe that the oral and anal phases and the Oedipal complex were the bases of human neurosis. Instead, Jung took a more holistic, right-brain, spiritual view of the human experience. He placed a syndrome such as depression at the heart of a person's engagement in the archetypal struggle for individuation. This struggle is seen by Jungians as a soul-journey whose imperative is freeing one's larger, genuine self from the false persona developed around the various wounds of childhood and the collective unconscious, in a sense birthing one's self into the world. The depressive's psychological pain might be viewed as labor pains, which are a natural and necessary accompaniment of any birth, including the birth of the self. In Jung's schema, depression is seen as the result of the unconscious but necessary process of the self tearing down the persona-life developed by the conforming ego.[14]

The Later 20th Century (1950–2000)

In the 1950s, both Edward Bibring and Edith Jackson built on Freud's psychological developmental theory. They emphasized the effect of loss of self-esteem as common to all types of depression. According to Bibring, self-esteem is based on a fixation at 1 of 3 Freudian stages. If one is fixated at the earliest oral phase of development, self-esteem is dependent on the need to be loved. As long as the possibility of being loved exists, depression is avoided. Fixation at the anal phase was presumed to create a belief that one's self-esteem depends on achieving a sense of control and power, while fixation at the Oedipal level creates the belief that one's self-esteem is dependent on the ability to be a loving person—to have one's love received. Helplessness and powerlessness develop when we are confronted with evidence that we cannot live up to our aspirations—we face the conflict between the ideal and the real. The loss of self-esteem is critical in this view. (Note that Jung's concept "What the ego idealizes, the Self tears down" is another perspective on this same process.) Life events are the triggers that transform diminished self-esteem into powerlessness and helplessness, and then into depression. This analytically based model implies that correction of underlying beliefs, generated in the developmental stages outlined by Freud, can treat the depression. Contrary to Freud's belief, however, the Bibring process is readily accessible to consciousness. Bibring's model can be seen as a bridge between the unconscious model of Freud and the next model of depression: the cognitive theory developed by the analytically trained Aaron Beck in the 1960s.

Beck[15] postulated that depression is the outcome of a variety of automatic and habitual distortions in thinking (e.g., all-or-nothing thinking, selective attention to the negative, fortune telling, catastrophizing—see *Feeling Good* by David Burns[16]), which lead quite naturally to depressive and anxious feelings. Feelings of any type are seen as the direct result of thinking, be it conscious, automatic (preconscious), or related to deeper schematic assumptions about life (unconscious). Beck identified what is now known as the cognitive triad of depression: negative views of the self, the future, and the world. He developed cognitive psychotherapy (now known as cognitive therapy) based on these observations. Cognitive therapy is a highly structured treatment in which negative automatic thoughts, patterned distortions of thinking, and underlying beliefs about life (schemas) are identified, tested for validity against reality, and then corrected. Building on the work of Martin Seligman (discussed below), the behavioral aspect of the treatment was later added for severely depressed individuals who could not benefit from cognitive work, and the treatment was renamed cognitive-behavioral therapy (CBT). Numerous studies have proven the efficacy of CBT in mild and moderate depression. (See Chapter 5, *Psychotherapy and Other Conventional Treatments*.)

Also in the 1960s, Seligman, a behaviorist, developed the first animal model of depression, which he termed learned helplessness. He published a full account of these breakthrough experiments in 1975.[17] In essence, Seligman proved that one can tolerate adversity and trauma as long as one has the ability to escape the aversive situation. However, when stress is inescapable, when a means of control is not available to attain one's essential goals (whether actual physical or psychic safety or essential self-esteem based on the need for love, power, or control, per Bibring), anxiety and agitation develop, quickly followed by a giving-up state: helplessness. Once helplessness is experienced, the possibility of helplessness becomes real. Helplessness and loss of control, as a state of being, have been learned, and the experience is permanently encoded in the brain, making the individual forever more vulnerable to seeing him or herself as lacking control, even when such control actually exists. In this animal model, helplessness is reversed behaviorally—that is, the situation is altered so that control and escape are indeed possible and the animal is actually forced to escape or take control. Some animals, and some people, strongly resist exercising control once they have experienced helplessness.

While the CBT and learned helplessness models were being developed and studied, Gerald Klerman and Myrna Weissman were formulating social theories of depression into a treatment model that was eventually outlined in a book called *Interpersonal Psychotherapy of Depression*.[18] Interpersonal psychotherapy (IPT) is based on the concept that depression can be conceptualized as a disturbance in interpersonal relationships, related to role changes, conflicts, and inadequate interpersonal skills.

Clinical Pearl:

In human terms, the CBT and learned helplessness models imply that the therapist must assess, in all people with depression, the source of the sense of helplessness (e.g., an alcoholic boss who controls one's promotion, a marital partner who is absent from the marriage, the loss of energy for living life due to a chronic medical condition, loss of function following an accident). In some cases, the person's view is accurate, and behavioral or situational change is indicated, while in other cases, the cognitive distortions are blurring the person's view of reality or possible ways of coping. Assessing these issues is paramount at the start of treatment.

The learned helplessness model and the CBT and IPT approaches to treatment are the psychotherapeutic foundation of today's conventional, nonpharmacological treatment of depression and should be familiar to anyone treating depression. As discussed in Chapter 5, CBT and IPT have been studied alone, against placebo, against medication, and in combination with medication. Researchers report nearly always that both therapies are as effective as medication in mild and moderate depression, although the evidence base for CBT is larger and stronger (see discussion in Chapter 5). There is also significant evidence that these 2 psychotherapies augment the benefits of medication and may target different symptom clusters when compared with medication.

Ban[19] posited that the history of psychopharmacology can be divided into 3 eras:

- The latter half of the 19th century
- The first half of the 20th century
- From 1950 forward (and ongoing)

Modern trends in psychopharmacology clearly have their roots in the 19th century, which saw the introduction of drugs such as morphine, bromine, and chloral hydrate. The early 20th century produced penicillin, whose effect on the delirium of syphilis fueled interest in drugs that could affect psychiatric symptoms.[20] This second psychopharmacological era also produced more than 2500 barbiturate preparations, of which "about 50 found a place in clinical practice as a hypnotic, sedative, anticonvulsant, general anesthetic, etc."[19] In the third era, the clinical use of lithium, chlorpromazine, reserpine, meprobamate, and the 2 seminal antidepressants imipramine and iproniazid catapulted psychopharmacology to the dominant place in psychiatric treatment that it occupies today. The increasing ability of physicians to control mental illness with drugs was a major factor in the unprecedented shift of treatment from psychiatric institutions to the community that occurred during this period. By the end of the 1970s, Ban stated, drug treatment had become the primary psychiatric modality.[20]

Many of the discoveries upon which modern psychopharmacology is based were serendipitous. Research on LSD, for example, focused on testing its ability to produce uterine contractions; during animal testing, the researcher Albert Hofmann was affected by the test substance in a way that triggered investigation of the psychomimetic effects of this powerful drug. Eventually, LSD was found to block peripheral serotonin receptors; the discovery contributed to the "revival of experimental psychiatry in the mid-1950s because it is reasonable to assume… that psychological symptoms that can be provoked by a drug, can also be abolished by drug action."[20] Other influential discoveries reinforced that assumption, and the development of the spectrophotofluorimeter "provided direct access to the detection of the biochemical changes responsible for… behavioral effects" through its ability to measure the concentration of cerebral monoamines and their metabolites.[19]

Observations that reserpine (an antihypertensive agent that was noted to deplete brain serotonin stores) seemed to trigger depression in a subset of hypertensive patients were seen as further indications that a biochemical basis for depression could be found.[21] The discovery that imipramine was therapeutic in depression resulted from a search for a treatment for schizophrenia.[20] The presentation in 1957 of research findings on imipramine, a tricyclic antidepressant that does not inhibit monoamine oxidase (MAO) but acts by inhibiting the reuptake of norepinephrine and serotonin, both peripherally and centrally, was contemporaneous with reports by another group of investigators on the drug iproniazid, which created a landmark shift in thinking that became known as the monoamine hypothesis of depression. The MAO hypothesis "proposes that the underlying biological or neuroanatomical basis for depression is a deficiency of central noradrenergic and/or serotonergic systems and that targeting this neuronal lesion with an antidepressant would tend to restore normal function in depressed patients."[21] Monoamine neurotransmitters provide important regulation of hypothalamic-pituitary-adrenal (HPA) activity; when HPA axis overactivity becomes chronic, it is linked to melancholic depression, characterized by hypercortisolism, adrenal hyperplasia, and abnormalities in negative feedback.[22]

Since the 1950s, "…various classes of antidepressive agents have been developed that act to increase the levels of monoamines within the synaptic cleft, either by inhibition of their degradation (MAO inhibitors) or by blockage of their reuptake"[21] (e.g., the tricyclics and selective serotonin reuptake inhibitors [SSRIs]). The development of the SSRIs was driven, in part, by a desire to reduce the remarkably unpleasant side effects of the tricyclic antidepressants and the potentially life-threatening food-medication interactions of the MAO inhibitors (MAOIs) that negatively impacted patient compliance with therapy. However, of all the antidepressant medications, only phenylzine[23] (an MAOI) was found to be consistently superior to other antidepressants in the treatment of atypical depression. A variety of antidepressant augmentation strategies have been researched and found somewhat effective (primarily lithium and thyroid—see Chapter 4).

From the psychiatrist's perspective, the advent of managed care in the 1990s has hastened the trend toward the psychopharmacological treatment of the depressive syndrome, marginalizing all but the most time-limited and structured therapies (CBT and IPT) for the treatment of depression. The treatment model came to be split between the psychiatrist, who knew little about the patient but prescribed the medications, and the therapist (often a psychologist or social worker), who knew more about the patient but had little influence on the medication regimen. Communication between these 2 parties was often less than optimal. Eventually, medication management of the mild and moderate depressives was moved (by the insurance and pharmaceutical companies) to the primary care physicians (family practitioners, obstetricians, and internists).

Other interesting and sometimes provocative views on the history of depression from the mid- to late 20th century are now beginning to emerge as scholarly retrospective reviews are written. One strong theme is that "depressive illness represents the final common pathway of several different pathogenetic processes... and is essentially the same whether the processes in question are biochemically, experientially, or behaviourally triggered."[24] However, Hirshbein made a persuasive argument that "depression as the illness that we know now is a twentieth-century phenomenon that... is framed by its social, cultural, professional and gender contexts."[25] She described the medicalization of depression in the 1950s and 1960s, pointing out that the use of antidepressants—medications that had an effect on patients who appeared depressed—had a strong effect on the modern diagnosis of depression as a disease entity ("the issue of how to understand and classify depression became tied up with the idea of being able to predict which patients would respond to medication"). ECT, even when used successfully, did not define a diagnosis, but use of antidepressants did seem to (although it is now known that antidepressants are helpful in multiple disorders including chronic pain syndromes, irritable bowel syndrome, generalized anxiety disorder, panic disorder, post-traumatic stress disorder, obsessive compulsive disorder, PMS, etc.). This is an odd twist on the history of depression and one that certainly reflects the pharmaceutical and insurance industry's growing influence on the practice of medicine in all its forms.

Hirshbein also discussed the feminization of depression, wherein the early research on antidepressants was done on women, who were disproportionately represented in hospital populations (perhaps for sociocultural reasons), leading to the development of theories, assessment tools, diagnostic classifications, and treatment approaches that—surprise!—led back to women. These events raise the possibility that depression in men might actually look different, and perhaps would be assessed and treated differently today, if we had comparable research on men. This view is somewhat supported by Rousseau,[1] who asserted that until the 18th century, "Madness had been primarily a male province ... ascribed to women only when the cults of sensibility strengthened from the mid-century. Madness was strong, noble, energetic; depression's female ancestors were weak, soft, ignoble, passive. Women were construed as primarily hysterical rather than mad...." As the concept of depression as an illness evolved to include notions of helplessness, passivity, and powerlessness, those coincided far more naturally with society's view of women than with its view of men, thus possibly leading to the disproportionate number of women diagnosed with and hospitalized for depressive disorders. The circularity in these issues is disturbing, to say the least. This feminization hypothesis is perhaps countered by the epidemiology, which indicates that rates of depression for males and females differ only during the reproductive years, when hormonal (and sociocultural) influences are strongest. (Perhaps the circularity of this argument implies that it is more useful to take a holistic, integrative approach to understanding depression, rather than a reductionistic approach.)

In nonpharmacologically driven medical hypotheses, multiple nutritional, hormonal, gastrointestinal, immunologic, genetic, and toxicological factors have been identified as contributing to or causing depression. (See Chapter 6, *Mechanisms and Interconnections within the Functional Medicine Matrix Model*.) Abram Hoffer pioneered the use of high doses of various nutrients to treat and even cure mental illness (orthomolecular psychiatry).[26] The methylation hypothesis of depression proposes that the methylation cycle (which utilizes folic acid, vitamin B12, S-adenosylmethionine, catechol-O-methyltransferase, and other factors) is central in the pathogenesis of many psychiatric disorders, including depression.

Clinical Pearl:

Folates and vitamin B12 have fundamental roles in central nervous system function at all ages, especially the methionine-synthase-mediated conversion of homocysteine to methionine, which is essential for both genomic and non-genomic methylation. Folic acid is a cofactor in production of tyrosine hydroxylase, the rate-limiting factor in dopamine synthesis, and in production of tryptophan hydroxylase, the rate-limiting step in serotonin synthesis.[27] Folate-deficient states have been associated with symptoms of depression, apathy, and impaired concentration,[28] and they have also been linked to a poor response to antidepressants.[29] In one study, the use of folic acid in augmentation of fluoxetine hydrochloride resulted in significantly improved response rates and reduced side effects.[30] It is presumed that the folate acts by increasing levels of catecholamines such as noradrenalin and dopamine.

The publication in 1980 of DSM-III represented a distillation and adoption of the modern affective disorders terminology, organized in the following schema:

- Major affective disorders
  - Bipolar disorders (mixed, manic, or depressed)
  - Major depressions (single episode or recurrent)
- Other specific affective disorders
  - Cyclothymic disorders
  - Dysthymic disorders (depressive neurosis)
- Atypical affective disorders
  - Atypical bipolar disorders
  - Atypical depressions

Etiology in DSM-III was used as a means of classification only if the evidence warranted it; otherwise, the groupings were made according to clinical, descriptive features. The diagnosis of endogenous depression has survived in clinical practice, and melancholia has resurfaced as a descriptor for the typically severe form of depression (although it was not used in DSM-III). It is important to note that these matters are not yet entirely settled, nor are they likely ever to be completely settled, as psychiatric/psychological theory and practice continue to evolve.

Current Prevailing Views

Classifications of Mood Disorders

Most professionals in the mental health field understand that the constantly shifting nature of psychiatric diagnostic criteria stems from several factors, including new research, changing culture, changing patterns of illness, changes in treatment, and changes in economic conditions. The search for clear boundaries between disorders is never ending, since all these parameters are in flux at one time or another and since the phenomenology of mood disorders is influenced by an alphabet soup of genetic and environmental factors, manifesting in infinite phenotypic expressions. While clusters of these phenotypes exist, they also shift over time and place. Ultimately, every depressive state will have its own unique fingerprint.

DSM-IV[31] (first published in 1994, with a text revision in 2000) differed from DSM-III in some important ways. For example, the atypical depression was included as a separate subtype of the Mood Disorders category (criteria included mood reactivity and at least 2 associated symptoms of hyperphagia, hypersomnolence, leaden fatigue, and rejection sensitivity as an enduring trait[32]). The clarification of this subtype as preferentially a MAOI-response state was made (in the circular way mentioned above) by including those patients who responded to the MAOIs.[32] However, as stated by Montgomery, "Whether antidepressants exert their action by correction of a monoamine deficiency or lesion or by upregulation or augmentation of intact monoamine systems is still a matter of some debate."[33]

Table 1.1—DSM-IV-TR Classification Schema for Mood Disorders[31]

- Mood Episodes
  - Major depressive episode
  - Manic episode
  - Mixed episode
  - Hypomanic episode
- Depressive Disorders
  - Major depressive disorder (one or more major depressive episodes comprising at least 2 weeks of depressed mood or loss of interest accompanied by at least 4 additional symptoms of depression)
  - Dysthymic disorder (at least 2 years of depressed mood for more days than not, accompanied by additional depressive symptoms that do not meet criteria for a major depressive episode)
  - Depressive disorder not otherwise specified (disorders with depressive features that do not meet the criteria for other categories)
- Bipolar I Disorders
  - Bipolar I disorder
  - Bipolar II disorder
  - Cyclothymic disorder
  - Bipolar disorder not otherwise specified
- Other Mood Disorders
  - Mood disorder due to [a specific general medical condition]
  - Substance-induced mood disorder
  - Mood disorder not otherwise specified

There are many specifiers that can be applied to a diagnosis, including degree of severity (mild, moderate, severe), presence or absence of psychotic features, partial or full remission, and—for depressive episodes—the presence of melancholic or atypical features. At the risk of oversimplifying the explanations provided in DSM-IV:

- The specifier *with melancholic features* is described as "loss of interest or pleasure in all, or almost all, activities or a lack of reactivity to usually pleasurable stimuli. The individual's depressed mood does not improve, even temporarily, when something good happens (Criterion A). In addition, at least 3 of the following symptoms are present: a distinct quality of the depressed mood, depression that is regularly worse in the morning, early morning awakening, psychomotor retardation or agitation, significant anorexia or weight loss, or excessive or inappropriate guilt (Criterion B)."[31]
- The essential characteristics of the specifier *with atypical features* are "mood reactivity [the capacity to be cheered up when presented with positive events] (Criterion A) and the presence of at least 2 of the following features (Criterion B): increased appetite or weight gain, hypersomnia, leaden paralysis, and a long-standing pattern of extreme sensitivity to perceived interpersonal rejection."[31] The differentiation of this subtype as preferentially a MAOI-response state seems to be supported by differences in HPA axis responsivity and clinical phenomenology, reflecting the (perhaps simplistic) hope of mainstream researchers that biochemical subtyping of depressive disorders will someday be possible.

In the late 20th and early 21st centuries, therefore, we find a nosology of depression that has eliminated the delusional disorders, defined a more narrow scope for the various types of depressive disease, and provided greater specificity for diagnostic work. The dominance of pharmacological approaches to treatment continues virtually unchecked, although a recent reduction in the use of antidepressants among children and teens following the black box warnings has been documented.[34, 35] Etiologic and therapeutic debates now focus on issues such as improving response rates via new biological treatments (modulation of HPA axis function, rTMS, and VNS); improving access to care; the roles of inflammation, infection, hormones, and neurogenesis; the interaction of genetics and environment (genomics); and the appropriate use of medication in childhood and adolescent depression. The importance of diet, environment, and lifestyle as antecedents, triggers, and mediators of depressive disorders is re-emerging as hypotheses about the myriad underlying pathways and multifactorial nature of the mood disorders are brought under scientific scrutiny (see Chapters 6 and 7).

Table 1.2—Primary Classes of Treatment

- Psychotherapy
    - Cognitive-behavioral therapy
    - Interpersonal therapy
- Pharmacotherapy
    - Selective serotonin reuptake inhibitors (citalopram, escitalopram oxalate, fluoxetine, fluvoxamine, paroxetine, sertraline)
    - Selective serotonin-norepinephrine reuptake inhibitors (venlafaxine, duloxetine)
    - Monoamine oxidase inhibitors (phenelzine, tranylcypromine, selegiline, moclobemide)
    - Tricyclics (amitriptyline, nortriptyline doxepin, imipramine, trimipramine, protriptyline, maprotiline clomipramine, amoxapine)
    - Others (buspirone, trazodone, reboxetine, mirtazapine, nefazodone, bupropion)
    - Lithium carbonate
    - Anticonvulsant mood stabilizers (lamotrigine, carbamazepine, oxcarbamazepine)
    - Antipsychotics (quetiapine)
    - Hormones (thyroid, estradiol patch, testosterone, DHEA)
- Electroconvulsive therapy
- Experimental treatments
    - Vagal nerve stimulation (VNS)
    - Repetitive transcranial magnetic stimulation (rTMS)

Integrative Summary

In a real sense, the history of depression is a mirror of the history of the ever-changing psychology of civilizations. The reader might feel bewildered by the history, and the authors, like those before them, might be inclined to hubris, pretending that we are, in this monograph, finally arriving at the *real* truth. We do not assert that; rather, we bring information about where things are at this point in time and how we got here.

Although much has changed over the millennia, some core issues—among them many that are critical to the functional medicine approach—are still deeply connected to our search for improved assessment, management, and prevention of depressive disorders. Modern theories about genomics have echoes in historical observations of genetic predispositions to melancholia. Constant sadness and feelings of helplessness and hopelessness are still core parts of the depressive experience. Identification in times past of upbringing and domestic troubles as influential factors appear today in concerns about the long-term effects of parental loss, exposure to violence or sexual abuse, and other early traumas, and are reflected in the current therapeutic approach of IPT. The spiritual dilemma of Job continues to echo in both the cognitive and depth psychological theories of the modern era.

So how does one integrate these seemingly disparate approaches? First, one must accept that depression is a psycho-spiritual-cultural-political-developmental-biological-genetic experience, affecting both the individual and the collective. Each of the epochs reviewed above has focused on particular aspects of this matrix, using its own language and beliefs as the lens through which it seeks understanding. Realizing this, if one takes a step back to see the whole, it is possible to envision the various subsystems interacting continuously with each other. Now it is the task of the healer to hold this perspective and use it to inform an approach to those who suffer with depression.

Any statement that we are finally arriving at some truth about depression would be nothing more than arrogance born of an ignorance of history. What we must accept, regardless of how uncomfortable not knowing can be, is that new conceptualizations, new information, and new paradigms will continue to make themselves known to us and that it is our duty as healers and scientists to remain forever open to new knowledge. As healers and scientists, we are destined to navigate the river of knowledge eternally, being surprised by new vistas with each twist and turn of our collective journey. When and how will the laws of quantum physics and the zero-point field impact our next advance in understanding of depression? How will our conceptualization and treatment options change when we begin to view the brain as a receiver of and integrator of multiple wave interference patterns in the quantum field between emotionally intimate individuals? What will truth look like if our culture moves from a reductionistic model to a systems model?

Ultimately, as any seasoned clinician will attest, healing will always remain something of a mystery, not least in our understanding and treatment of depression. Paradoxically, this mystery, while limiting our efficacy and control, will highlight our need for faith and keep us forever humble and curious, as we should be, in our search for understanding of depression.

References

1. Rousseau G. Depression's forgotten genealogy: notes towards a history of depression. *Hist Psychiatry*. 2000;11:71-106.
2. Kraepelin E. *Dementia Praecox*. Edinburgh, Scotland: E.S. Livingstone; 1919.
3. Bleuler E. *Dementia Praecox and the Group of Schizophrenias*. New York: International Universities Press; 1950.
4. Jackson SA. *Melancholia and Depression: From Hippocratic Times to Modern Times*. New Haven and London: Yale University Press; 1986.
5. Gorman J. Maimonides, 1135-1204. *Am J Psychiatry*. 2001;158:376.
6. Bloch S. Moses Maimonides' contribution to the biopsychosocial approach in clinical medicine. *Lancet*. 2001;358:829-832.
7. Brieger P, Marneros A. Dysthymia and cyclothymia: historical origins and contemporary development. *J Affect Disord*. 1997;45:117-126.
8. Burton R. *The Anatomy of Melancholy*. New York, NY: The New York Review of Books; 2001.
9. Ehrenreich B. How we learned to stop having fun. *Guardian*. 2007.
10. Johnson S. *A Dictionary of the English Language: An Anthology*. Crystal D, ed. London: Penguin Classics; 2006.
11. Laffey P. Psychiatric therapy in Georgian Britain. *Psychol Med*. 2003;33:1285-1297.
12. Freud S. Mourning and Melancholia. In: Gay P, ed. *The Freud Reader*. New York, N.Y.: W.W. Norton & Company, Inc.:584-588.
13. Gabbard GO, Gunderson JG, Fonagy P. The place of psychoanalytic treatments within psychiatry. *Arch Gen Psychiatry*. 2002;59:505-510.
14. Zimberoff D, Hartman D. Attachment, Detachment, Nonattachment: Achieving Synthesis. *Journal of Heart-Centered Therapies*. 2002;5:3-94.
15. Beck AT. *Depression*. New York: Hoeber; 1967.
16. Burns DD. *Feeling Good*. New York, NY: Avon Books; 1999.
17. Seligman MEP. *Helplessness: On Depression, Development, and Death*. San Francisco: Freeman; 1975.
18. Klerman GL, Weissman MM, Rounsaville BJ, Chevron ES. *Interpersonal Psychotherapy of Depression*. New York: Basic; 1984.
19. Ban TA. Pharmacotherapy of mental illness--a historical analysis. *Prog Neuropsychopharmacol Biol Psychiatry*. 2001;25:709-727.
20. Ban TA. The role of serendipity in drug discovery. *Dialogues Clin Neurosci*. 2006;8:335-344.
21. Hirschfeld RM. History and evolution of the monoamine hypothesis of depression. *J Clin Psychiatry*. 2000;61 Suppl 6:4-6.
22. Dinan TG, Scott LV. Anatomy of melancholia: focus on hypothalamic-pituitary-adrenal axis overactivity and the role of vasopressin. *J Anat*. 2005;207:259-264.
23. Stewart JW, Thase ME. Treating DSM-IV Depression with Atypical Features. *J Clin Psychiatry*. 2007;68:e10.
24. Cooper B. Sylvia Plath and the depression continuum. *J R Soc Med*. 2003;96:296-301.
25. Hirshbein LD. Science, gender, and the emergence of depression in American psychiatry, 1952-1980. *J Hist Med Allied Sci*. 2006;61:187-216.
26. Hoffer A. Orthomolecular psychiatry. *Biol Psychiatry*. 1979;14:453-454.
27. Lombard J. Neurotransmitters: a functional medicine approach to neuropsychiatry. In: Jones DS, ed. *Textbook of Functional Medicine*. Gig Harbor, WA: Institute for Functional Medicine; 2005:638-644.
28. Alpert JE, Fava M. Nutrition and depression: the role of folate. *Nutr Rev*. 1997;55:145-149.
29. Coppen A, Bolander-Gouaille C. Treatment of depression: time to consider folic acid and vitamin B12. *J Psychopharmacol*. 2005;19:59-65.
30. Coppen A, Bailey J. Enhancement of the antidepressant action of fluoxetine by folic acid: a randomised, placebo controlled trial. *J Affect Disord*. 2000;60:121-130.
31. *Diagnostic and Statistical Manual of Mental Disorders, Fourth Edition, Text Revision (DSM-IV-TR)*. Arlington, VA: American Psychiatric Association; 2000.
32. Davidson JR. A history of the concept of atypical depression. *J Clin Psychiatry*. 2007;68 Suppl 3:10-15.
33. Montgomery S. Understanding depression and its treatment: Restoration of chemical balance or creation of conditions promoting recovery? *J Clin Psychiatry*. 2000;61:3.
34. Gibbons RD, Brown CH, Hur K, et al. Early evidence on the effects of regulators' suicidality warnings on SSRI prescriptions and suicide in children and adolescents. *Am J Psychiatry*. 2007;164:1356-1363.
35. Olfson M, Marcus SC, Druss BG. Effects of Food and Drug Administration warnings on antidepressant use in a national sample. *Arch Gen Psychiatry*. 2008;65:94-101.

Chapter 2

The Cultural Context of Depression

Depression in Western Culture

Depression occurs worldwide and affects all cultures and members of all ethnic groups. As discussed in Chapter 3, *Epidemiology and Public Health Impact*, the world is currently experiencing epidemic levels of depression. In the United States, the projected lifetime risk for major depressive disorder at age 75 was 23.2%—nearly a quarter of the U.S. population.[1] The World Health Organization estimates that depression affects about 121 million people worldwide and is the leading cause of disability (as measured in years living with disability [YLDs]),[2] accounting for almost 12% of all disability.[3]

As practitioners, as patients, and as members of the human community, we cannot fully assess the nature of depression without addressing the context (culture, community, family) within which it occurs. Although most of this monograph will focus on assessment and treatment for individual patients, to discuss the rising incidence and prevalence of depression (see Chapter 3) without exploring the cultural medium within which this phenomenon is occurring would be to cover only part of the story. The specific context for most of what we have written is primarily Western culture, communities, and families, but that does not mean the information lacks applicability across other cultures—the globalization of culture is an ongoing and accelerating process.

Western culture, according to Richard Tarnas,[4] has evolved over the last few millennia in such a manner that modern humankind has become alienated, disoriented, and unconscious. Despite the very significant advances afforded by developments in knowledge and technology, and despite the wealth accumulated in the world's top economies, we cannot help but see the dark side of modern culture in the form of the global displacement, disempowerment, illness, and death of millions of people and thousands of communities through wars, epidemic diseases, ecological disequilibrium (e.g., climate change), and economic disparities.

The Western worldview has been primarily that we live in an inanimate universe with other life forms that are essentially unconscious. We are unique in the universe and, as a corollary to that, we are alone and superior. We believe that science is the only valid way of knowing. In a neuroanatomical sense, we have overprivileged the prefrontal cortex and left hemisphere of the brain. We grapple with what seems to be an inescapable conclusion: we live in an essentially meaningless, purely physical, random world, in which we are intrinsically separate from others, separate from nature, and separate from a creator (if we believe in one). This is the context within which depression has grown dramatically in incidence and prevalence. If worldviews create worlds, as asserted by cognitive therapy, the leading psychotherapy of depression, then we must wonder what it is about the Western worldview that has created a context within which depression has become a major cause of disability and suffering.

The physical world that has fed the culture of depression is the densely populated Westernized city, in which we are paradoxically both closer to and more apart from others. It is made of concrete, steel, glass, plastic, and asphalt. Most of us breathe hydrocarbon-polluted air, eat nutritionally vacuous (or even harmful) food (*trans*-fatty acids, pesticides, and herbicides), and drink plasticized bottled water (phthalates). If we are fortunate, we may have a mountain or ocean or forest retreat from the man-made environment. If we are less affluent, we may make special trips to reconnect with nature at the local zoo or botanical gardens. But for most of us, nature is absent from our daily lives. We have become estranged from an important and deep aspect of the world into which all species were born and within which all evolved. We do not, in a personal sense, understand nature as Thoreau came to, when he was at Walden Pond. We see time passing in the faces of our loved ones or in the mirror, but we do not experience the naturalness of the passage of time via a slowly changing landscape. We have lost the mirroring experience and sense of perspective which the natural world provides. And so we are left with a tremendous existential aloneness and anxiety about the strangeness of death, which seems quite disconnected from life and therefore fails to inform our lives with meaning and value. We cannot be chaperoned through the stages of our lives by nature. And so we cling to youth, attempting to freeze time.

In our constructed, urban environments, where there is no inherent meaning and no dialogue with nature, we seek solace in the physical. We buy and consume far more than we need. We work ever harder to buy and consume ever more, in order to experience short-lived feelings of satisfaction or achievement or safety. In the effort to produce, earn, purchase and consume, we fill our lives with work and often meaning-free activities, becoming alienated from our families, coworkers, friends, and communities. The capitalistic ethos seems to have replaced a commitment to a higher purpose. The observation by Alexis de Tocqueville 165 years ago in his great tome *Democracy in America* that "the business of America is business" represents a view that has spread throughout the world, bringing for many people ever greater wealth, absence of acute infectious diseases, and freedom from harsh physical labor, but also contributing to the rapidly rising incidence of chronic physical illness, as well as emotional and spiritual pain.

It is indeed tragic that as a society we allow ourselves to remain largely unconscious about the issues raised above and about their effects on other cultures and on our planet. In the last 90 years, 2 world wars, multiple holocausts, constant environmental degradation and human exposure to toxic chemicals, threatened nuclear annihilation, and now a massive global ecological imbalance are in our consciousness as individuals; yet, as political parties, as families, communities, professions, governments, and as a culture, we are willing to be silent about the clear evidence that, in many ways, our current approach to human existence is failing.

To circle around to the topic at hand—if one is living in a fundamentally imbalanced (i.e., insane) culture, is it surprising that greater and greater numbers of individuals are presenting with depression? Should we be so myopically focused on the individual? Can and should the individual carry the full burden for recovery from depression? Is not this focus on the individual—one might even say, this cult of personal responsibility—part of the reductionistic thinking that has helped to create the problem?

On a collective level, higher numbers of depressed, nonfunctioning individuals are already producing a negative feedback loop within this culture, via the growth of chronic disease and excessive healthcare costs and via reduced viability of the individual, the family unit, and therefore the community—all known sequelae of depression. If we can learn about and understand the links between the brain and the immune system and between diet and mood, shouldn't we also seriously investigate the links between the culture and individual behavior, between the stresses of Western psychology and the craving for something to satisfy the inner emptiness? Is there not perhaps a link between this yearning and the obsessive purchase of material goods and the excessive intake of (nutrient-poor) food?

Depression in Other Cultures

The presenting picture of depressive diseases varies not only with the times (see Chapter 1, *History and Prevailing Views*), but also with the culture. In Asian cultures, for example, patients with depression will often present with somatic complaints because "the whole idea of illness in Eastern cultures is based on physical illness... either you have physical illness or you're not sick."[5] Culture influences how a patient experiences an illness such as depression (symptoms), how he/she presents (signs), and how he or she feels about it. For example, "Many depressed Chinese people do not report feeling sad, but rather express boredom, discomfort, feelings of inner pressure, and symptoms of pain, dizziness, and fatigue."[6] Mental illness may be seen as evidence of bad genes, a stain on the family's heritage, and thus an obstacle for the children in making good marriages.[5] In Ayurvedic medicine, the existence of a "winter depression"—comparable to seasonal affective disorder—is recognized,[7] but it is seen as a result of certain physical imbalances and not as mental illness.

It is beyond the scope of this monograph to explore cultural variations in the experience and presentation of depressive disorders, but it is very important that clinicians inform themselves because "culture influences the experience of symptoms, the idioms used to report them, decisions about treatment, doctor-patient interactions, the likelihood of outcomes such as suicide, and the practices of professionals."[6]

Summary

Ultimately, it is likely that a really significant reduction in the incidence and prevalence of depression on a public health scale will not come from antidepressants, individual psychotherapy, or from fish oil. It will come from a reconnection of the individual with the family, the community, a purposeful culture, and a dialogue with nature and meaning. This will require a rebalancing of the individualistic, domination-oriented culture (in which reason and logic are the only ways of knowing and wealth represents power and success) with the holistic, interactive, and participatory approach to life. We as human beings need a balance of both to thrive. Socioeconomic and political efforts to incorporate such an integrated view of ourselves, the world, and our future as a species are the therapy that this culture requires if we are to stem the rising tide of depression.

Just as in the Jewish culture, where the *Vidui* states that the collective community is responsible for the well-being and good behavior of the individual, so too must society and culture be held accountable for their roles in the mental health and well-being of individuals. Thus, providers of treatment to depressed patients must also pay attention to these critical issues.

References

1. Kessler RC, Berglund P, Demler O, Jin R, Merikangas KR, Walters EE. Lifetime prevalence and age-of-onset distributions of DSM-IV disorders in the National Comorbidity Survey Replication. *Arch Gen Psychiatry.* 2005;62:593-602.
2. WHO Initiative on Depression in Public Health. http://www.who.int/mental_health/management/depression/depressioninph/en/. Accessed March 10, 2008.
3. Palpant RG, Steimnitz R, Bornemann TH, Hawkins K. The Carter Center Mental Health Program: Addressing the public health crisis in the field of mental health through policy change and stigma reduction. *Preventing Chronic Disease.* 2006;3:1-6.
4. Tarnas R. *The Passion of the Western Mind: Understanding the Ideas that Have Shaped Our World View*: Ballantine Books; Reprinted 1993.
5. Medscape.com. Eastern vs Western Perspectives on Depression: An Expert Interview with James C.-Y. Chou, MD. http://www.medscape.com/viewarticle/501758. Accessed March 10, 2008.
6. Kleinman A. Culture and depression. *N Engl J Med.* 2004;351:951-953.
7. Ayurveda Holistic Community. Ayurveda Regime for Winter Depression. http://www.ayurvedahc.com/articlelive/articles/183/1/-Ayurveda-regime-for-winter-depression/Page1.html. Accessed April 5, 2007.

Chapter 3

Epidemiology and Public Health Impact

The Epidemiology of Depression

The epidemiological picture of (unipolar) depression has been changing over the past several decades. Shifts have occurred in age-related factors, prevalence, and projected lifetime risk (the increased prevalence we see today echoes the epidemic increase in depression in England in the 1600s, referred to in Chapter 1). These shifts do not appear to be related to better assessment and diagnostic capacities; rather, they are related to an unmasking of genetic predispositions induced by increased burdens on any of the systems known to contribute to mood disorders (e.g., early trauma, psychological learned helplessness and defeat, sociocultural isolation, economic deprivation, spiritual alienation, nutritional insufficiencies, hormonal dysregulation, increased immune and inflammatory burden). For clinicians, this means that *every patient's individual pathway toward depression needs to be explored and fully understood.*[1] For policy makers and public health experts, there are other implications.

As with all epidemiological studies, the information can be applied with some confidence to very large groups of people, but with less reliability to the individual patient. Nonetheless, understanding the epidemiology can change clinician awareness about risk factors (e.g., membership in a high-risk group, life event antecedents, comorbid conditions) and can offer insights into the context within which depression occurs for the individual patient.

Although large studies have reported different prevalence figures for major depressive disorder (MDD),[2, 3] the trend since the early 1980s is clearly upward for both current (i.e., 12-month) and lifetime disorder—from 3.5% and 5.9% in the National Institute of Mental Health Epidemiologic Catchment Area Study of the early 1980s[4] to 8.6% and 14.9% in the National Comorbidity Survey (1990-1992),[5] 5.28% and 13.23% in the National Epidemiologic Survey on Alcoholism and Related Conditions (NESARC, 2001-02),[2] and 6.6% and 16.2% in the National Comorbidity Survey Replication (NCS-R, also 2001-02).[3] Over the years, diagnostic criteria and instruments have changed, survey age groupings have differed, and societal attitudes toward depression have relaxed; all these shifts (and many methodological issues and study limitations) make exact comparisons of the data technically challenging. The trend, however, is not disputed, nor are most of the major epidemiological factors.

Several consistent and well-documented associations have been reported. Taken as a whole, the associations below confirm that depression is a complex disorder, with multiple genetic and environmental influences interacting to create the ultimate outcome.

- MDD is the most prevalent mental health condition among the DSM-IV[6] disorders; the projected lifetime risk at age 75 was 23.2%, nearly a quarter of the U.S. population. The lifetime prevalence of having *any* DSM-IV disorder was 46.4%, nearly half the U.S. population.[7] More than 19 million people in the United States alone suffer from depression, but only one third actually receive treatment.[8]

- Both NESARC and NCS-R found that depression is considerably more common in women than men, a consistent finding over many years.[2, 3] Lifetime prevalence of MDD for women may be as much as twice that for men.[9, 10] This appears to be particularly true during the reproductive years, following which the differences tend to disappear.[10] Studies have found that the greatest risk for women is during times of fluctuating estrogen (e.g., perimenopause[11-13] and postpartum[14]). NESARC also reported that women get treatment with greater frequency than men.[2]

- Compared to Caucasians, Native Americans have the highest odds ratio (1.5), while Asians (0.6), Hispanics (0.6), and African-Americans (0.7) have much lower odds ratios.[2]

- The risk for MDD is low until adolescence, and then the curves for all age groups studied rise sharply,[3] with mean age at onset reported in NESARC as 30.4 years and in NCS-R as 30 years.[7] NESARC also reported a mean age at first treatment of 33.5, indicating a considerable lag between initial onset and first treatment.[2] Lifetime incidence in those 60 and older is lower than the younger age groups.[2, 3, 7, 15]

- MDD is strongly associated with alcohol- and drug-related disorders, with smoking, and with anxiety and personality disorders.[2, 3]

- Unemployment (whether because of disability, homemaker status, or other reasons), poverty, and education of less than 12 years are notable socioeconomic risk factors.[3]

- Genetic risk factors for MDD have been identified.[1, 16] A meta-analysis of the genetic epidemiology of major depression[1] estimated the heritability in the range of 31% to 42%. This meta-analysis determined that, while most of this association appears to be a result of genetics when populations are studied, both genetics and environment are critical etiologic factors for the individual patient, a result supported elsewhere.[17]

- High levels of lifetime adversity are causally related to both depression and anxiety, even when traumatic events occurred years or even decades earlier.[18] Among the most traumatic experiences studied are sexual abuse and physical violence (both direct experience and witnessing).[18, 14] Parental death, psychopathology, and substance abuse are also key risk factors,[18] as is parental divorce.[19, 20] Women are more strongly affected by early parental divorce, the effects of which are measurable into adulthood.[20, 21]

Virtually all epidemiological studies of depression report a strong association with significant impairment in activities of daily living (role impairment); NCS-R reported the impairment in social role to be greater than impairment in the work role.[3] Thus, the role of inadequately treated depression as a contributor to the rising rates of divorce, adolescent depression, substance abuse, ADD, etc. must be investigated. Both NCS-R and NESARC report that the degree of role impairment is strongly associated with symptom severity.[2, 3] NESARC found that "almost half the respondents with MDD thought about suicide or wanted to die."[2]

Overall mortality risks are higher for people with depression and depressive symptoms,[8, 22, 23] although to what degree is not yet clear. A 2006 review of death certificates,[24] for example, uncovered major omissions of psychiatric conditions from cause of death information, perhaps leading to significant underestimates of the contributions of depression and other psychiatric disorders to mortality. It is also unclear whether depression is an independent risk factor for mortality. As discussed below (see *Public Health Impact of Depression*), depression is both a major contributor to, and a common result of, many other chronic health conditions; it is possible that morbidity, disability, and lifestyle factors of comorbid conditions can explain most of the association of depression with mortality.[25-27] The research is strongest for an association between depression and mortality in patients who are already part of the psychiatric population and in patients with heart disease,[28] rather than as an independent predictor for previously healthy people.[26] Among psychiatric patients with mood disorders, however, depression is the disorder most strongly associated with suicide.[29]

Despite these powerful indications of the urgent need for treatment, *a serious lack of treatment frequency and adequacy was found.* Considering that symptoms and symptom severity among MDD patients in primary and specialty outpatient care do not differ substantially, this is a stunning indictment of the entire mental health system. NESARC found lack of treatment to be particularly marked in men, only 50.5% of whom received any treatment at all; 65.5%

of women had sought treatment within the year of the interview (12-month group), but the definition of *treatment* was not correlated in any way with effectiveness. NSC-R found that 57.3% of all respondents with 12-month MDD received some type of treatment; however, "no more than 21.6% of all respondents with 12-month MDD... received adequate treatment in the year of the interview."[3] The authors defined *adequate treatment* according to recommendations from evidence-based treatment guidelines.[i] Of even greater concern is that among individuals with very severe and severe 12-month MDD, only 39.1% and 24.6%, respectively, received adequate treatment.[3]

The problem is not confined to the United States. A 2007 examination of data collected by the World Health Organization (WHO) in 24 countries and by INSERM in France "revealed that only 54% to 58% of depressed patients were recognized as 'psychiatric cases' by their general practitioner and only 15% to 26% were given a specific diagnosis of depression.[30] Even when cases were recognized, treatment was frequently inappropriate."

To summarize, the epidemiology of depression brings to life the pervasive and disabling impact of this condition, highlighting the critical need for improved identification and treatment of patients with all ranges of depressive symptomatology. However, it is also urgent that we effectively integrate our understanding of the mechanisms, conditions, and effects that contribute to the broad picture painted above into a new treatment paradigm. *Reliance on a paradigm that is essentially restricted to medication and therapy has proved inadequate for most of the people affected by and treated for depression.*

Public Health Impact of Depression

Statistics alone cannot convey the personal and familial impact of living with the mental and emotional pain of depression, but statistics can help to establish greater awareness of the global public health impact of depression and to elevate the priority for identifying and treating this pervasive and debilitating disease, whether it presents as a primary or a comorbid condition.

Depression-Associated Disability

Despite the perception that most of the world's mortality and morbidity are caused by infectious disease and other somatic conditions, mental illness ranks as the top cause of disability-adjusted life years (DALYs)[ii] worldwide and is the second leading cause even in low-income and lower-middle-income countries.[31] "By 2020, major depression is expected to be second only to ischemic heart disease as a cause of disability."[32] WHO estimates that depression affects about 121 million people worldwide and is the leading cause of disability (as measured in years living with disability [YLDs]),[33] accounting for almost 12% of all disability.[34] Already, WHO reports that depression is the second-leading cause of DALYs in the 15–44 age group for both men and women combined, while "between 10 and 15% of the child and adolescent population has some symptoms of depression."[35]

A recent investigation of disability-associated retirement found that "anxiety and depression were robust predictors of disability pension awards in general, *even when disability pensions awarded for any mental disorder were excluded* [emphasis added]."[36] This finding, if replicated, would indicate that depression-associated disability is actually underestimated.

---

[i] Minimal treatment adequacy was defined by the researchers as "receiving either (1) at least 4 outpatient visits with any type of physician for pharmacotherapy that included use of either an antidepressant or mood stabilizer for a minimum of 30 days or (2) at least 8 outpatient visits with any professional in the specialty mental health sector for psychotherapy lasting a mean of at least 30 minutes."

[ii] The sum of years of potential life lost due to premature mortality and the years of productive life lost due to disability. [Murray CJL, Lopez AD. Evidence-based health policy—lessons from the Global Burden of Disease Study. *Science*. 1996;274:740-743.]

The Cost of Depression

The economic impact of depression can be perceived in myriad ways: as a driver for increasing costs within the healthcare system, as a cost to employers in lost productive time both at work and in absenteeism, as a relatively untreated comorbidity with many of the most common chronic diseases, as a risk factor for the development of chronic disease, and, not least, in terms of human suffering and loss of life. (Suicide, which accounts for 49.1% of intentional violent deaths worldwide,[34] is fueled by depression.)

Consider the following facts:

- U.S. workers with depression cost employers an estimated $44 billion per year in lost productive time (LPT), an excess of $31 billion per year compared with peers without depression, not including the labor costs associated with short- and long-term disability.[37] Many aspects of job performance are impaired by depression, and the impact persists even after symptoms improve.[38]
- The cost of health care is rising rapidly in the United States, driven in great part by our increasing dependence on prescription drugs,[iii] the most common and well-researched treatment for depression (and, of course, for most other chronic diseases, as well). If this trend continues uncorrected, the economic burden is likely to become untenable within the next decade.
- Children born today represent the first generation whose life expectancy may actually be less than that of preceding generations, a dire situation that is being fueled by the rise in obesity and obesity-related conditions,[39] which are comorbid with depression and are drivers for many other common and costly chronic diseases such as diabetes and heart disease. In fact, most office visits today to primary care practitioners concern chronic, not acute, diseases.[40]
- Most common chronic medical conditions have well-documented reciprocal relationships with depression. Untreated (or unsuccessfully treated) depression is a significant contributor to the economic impact and the human suffering involved in chronic disease, and it also makes successful treatment of medical conditions (as differentiated, diagnostically if not functionally, from mental disease) less likely and more costly.[32]
- As our population ages, the effects of these trends are likely to be exacerbated because depression in the elderly is not only common, but it adversely affects physical and cognitive functioning, generating a need for extra care that was estimated in 2004 to be the equivalent of $9 billion per year.[41]

Depression as a Comorbid Condition

Depression is associated very strongly with comorbidity,[42] making it urgent that practitioners understand the degree to which it may be a risk factor for, or a concomitant condition with, **any** chronic disease. Most of us can easily identify the most common chronic diseases in the United States (and most of the developed world): heart disease, cancer, diabetes, asthma/allergy, obesity, hypertension, stroke. These will be uppermost in any clinician's mind when evaluating suffering patients. What is less clear is whether clinicians will recognize that every one of those diseases has a strong association with depression,[40] and that health-related quality of life can be further impaired by that association, as measured by the decline of physical and mental function.[43]

Not only is depression associated with increased prevalence of chronic disease, but chronic diseases can exacerbate symptoms of depression. We will examine the complex relationship of depression to some of the most common and costly chronic diseases, focusing first on diabetes and then on cardiovascular and cerebrovascular conditions, which have a very extensive literature to draw upon. Further examples of other chronic diseases associated with depression will highlight the importance of screening for, preventing, and treating depression in all patients who seek care for medical conditions, but they are not the only conditions where such an approach is critical. The linkages among socioeconomic and cultural factors affecting both mind and body are dynamic, reverberating, and multidirectional; effective care for all chronic disease must address all aspects of the problem to achieve better outcomes. The following sections do not provide a comprehensive review of all diseases and conditions associated with depression; they should serve, rather, as a wake-up call for clinicians to routinely (and effectively) screen for depression in all patients with chronic disease and, if identified, to treat (or refer) appropriately.

We should keep in mind 2 major limitations of many of the studies on depression comorbidities and effects of treatment:

1. They fail to differentiate between the 2 well-established and very different types of major depression (typical/hypercortisolemic/hypernoradrenergic/melancholic and atypical/hypocortisolemic/hyponoradrenergic/reactive).
2. They fail to distinguish between those who fully respond to the antidepressant treatment and those who are partial or nonresponders: "Although over 90% of depressed patients will eventually 'respond' to one or a combination of different drugs, up to half of these will never [fully] remit, and for those who do, up to 30% do not remain well in the first 18 months following remission."[44] This finding translates to approximately one-third full responders and two-thirds non- or partial responders.

These distinctions are critical for accurately determining treatment effects. For example, in order to determine accurately whether HgA1c is elevated by comorbid depression and reduced by depression treatment, one must compare *only* complete antidepressant responders (where presumably much of the underlying pathophysiology has been corrected) to untreated depressive diabetics. Despite these limitations, however, associations and trends have emerged from the literature, and it can be very useful to review them.

Depression and diabetes — Patients with type 2 diabetes have twice the rate of depression as the general population,[32, 45-48] and the coexistence of both conditions is responsible for an increase in mortality that is greater than that due to having either condition alone.[49] One study reported a 1.3-fold increase compared to people with only diabetes, a 2-fold increase compared to people with only depression, and a 2.5-fold increase compared to people who have neither condition.[46] There have been many studies over the last several decades examining the relationship between depression and diabetes—in fact, this may be the most well-researched comorbidity. Interesting hypotheses have appeared, been tested, and been confirmed or dropped. The ongoing work has contributed to the depression and chronic disease literature as a whole, and even more importantly (certainly for the diabetic patient), it has identified a critical need for improving outcomes in diabetic patients by screening for and competently treating depression.

For clinicians who see patients with diabetes, screening for and treating depression should be a consistent strategy, but unfortunately that is not the case. Most patients with chronic medical illness are treated in primary, rather than specialty, settings, which can adversely affect both the competence and frequency of assessment and treatment for depression.[50, 51] For example, a 1998 study reported that "approximately two thirds of patients who have both diabetes and major depression do not receive antidepressant treatment, in part because their physicians tend to attribute their depression to poorly controlled or advancing diabetes."[52] Another study reported that "depression is recognized and treated appropriately in fewer than 25% of depressed diabetic patients."[47] Barriers to high-quality care for these comorbid conditions may include "suboptimal recognition; inconsistent treatment with lack of close follow-up and monitoring; and organizational barriers."[53] These deficits may stem, at least in part, from a discrepancy between perceived and actual ability to recognize common mental disorders.[54] If clinicians believe that they are already adequately skilled, they will not seek training to improve their accuracy.

Within the last few years, some clarity has begun to emerge about causality. It is now fairly well established that depression is a significant and independent risk factor for the development of diabetes[46, 55]; whether this is because of disturbances in the hypothalamic-pituitary-adrenal (HPA) axis that increase insulin resistance and weight gain (which, in turn, raise the risk of diabetes), or because of changes in the metabolism of certain neurotransmitters (alterations that are also seen in diabetes), or because of the impact of psychosocial factors (reduced quality of self-care)—or possibly some combination of all these factors—is not yet known.[49, 56, 57] A very pertinent study published in 2008[58] found that "Nondepressed women and men with metabolic syndrome at baseline were twice as likely to have depressive symptoms at follow-up...." Metabolic syndrome, with its high degree of insulin resistance, apparently shows the same type of comorbidity with depression as diabetes. We do not have to know the precise underlying mechanisms, or their proportional contributions, to extrapolate that the rapid rise in the prevalence of diabetes in the United States[49] must be, at least partially, a reflection of the increasing prevalence of depression.

For most patients with type 2 diabetes, the diagnosis of depression precedes that of diabetes, making it unlikely that primary causality for most patients proceeds from diabetes to depression.[56] However, in type 1 diabetes, depression typically follows the diagnosis, which is usually made much earlier in life.[56] Efforts to identify the factors that differentiate the relationship of the 2 types of diabetes to depression are under way, but no consensus has yet emerged. Although the causality direction may not typically move from type 2 diabetes to depression, there is considerable evidence about the worsening of depression in the presence of multiple complications of diabetes and as a result of perceived illness intrusiveness and loss of social support.[32, 56] There is also a long history of evidence indicating that the presence of depression adversely impacts the management of diabetes.[50, 57, 59, 60] Causality aside, therefore, it is correct to say that the presence of diabetes does affect the course and prevalence of depression. It would also be accurate to say that the relationship between diabetes and depression is bidirectional, synergistic, and very influential over time in the course of both conditions and in ultimate patient outcomes.

A very interesting study testing the direction of causality between metabolic syndrome and depression was published in 2007.[58] The authors evaluated a large group of patients for both metabolic syndrome and depression in 1998 and again 7 years later. They found that nondepressed individuals with metabolic syndrome at baseline were twice as likely to have depressive symptoms 7 years later, with lipid levels contributing most strongly to the odds ratio.

Among the many effects that living with both depression and diabetes has on patients are the following:

- "Among people with diabetes mellitus, those with depression have higher levels of work disability or overall functional disability (i.e., non-work-related) compared with those without depression."[32] The work-related disability involves both the inability to be present in the workplace and the inability to perform tasks while there.
- Effective management of diabetes is extremely dependent on competent self-care; as much as 95% of diabetes management is actually handled by the patient.[50] Tellingly, patients with comorbid depression and diabetes have greater difficulty adhering to dietary recommendations, carrying through on exercise plans, monitoring blood glucose, and taking medications as prescribed.[50]
- Diabetic patients with depression have poorer glycemic control (primarily in type 1 diabetes[60, 61]) and an increased incidence of micro- and macrovascular complications, both key indicators of a far more serious course of illness.[53]
- The presence of both conditions has also been associated with poorer mental functioning and lower self-perceived health status, both contributing to a significantly decreased quality of life.[32]
- Patients with comorbid diabetes and depression are much higher utilizers of the healthcare system and thus generate higher costs.[46, 50]

Reviewing the extensive literature on associations, causality, and prevalence might lead one to wonder whether there have been equally far-reaching investigations of the effects of treating depression in diabetic patients. Issues concerning treatment effects have begun to be reported on in some depth, but the questions still far outstrip the answers. Since a substantial portion of the present monograph will be devoted to a discussion of treatments for depression, including a broadening of the treatment armamentarium to include functional medicine approaches, we will not spend a great deal of time examining this particular aspect of treatment. However, a brief look at a few promising interventions in the depression-diabetes pairing raises many points of interest.

An important meta-analysis in 2000 suggested that effective treatment for depression was likely to increase the proportion of patients "in good control from 41 to 58% in a diabetic population"[59]—a considerable potential benefit. (It should be noted that, unless otherwise stated, treatment in these studies consists primarily and often exclusively of antidepressant medications.) A few studies have reported improvements in such indicators as glycemic control as a result of treating depression in diabetic patients,[55, 62, 63] although others have found a worsening impact on glycemic control.[64] In general, the contradictory findings are thought to be the result of using different drugs. The Pathways Study, a randomized controlled trial on collaborative care for patients with diabetes and depression, has resulted in only a few publications so far, but some intriguing results have been reported. The study utilized a collaborative care model, defined as a multimodal intervention utilizing a care manager (nurses with special training in both medical and mental health management of diabetes and depression[51]) working in concert with a psychiatrist, a psychologist, and a primary care physician.[57] The researchers found that this enhanced treatment model had a significant positive effect on symptoms of depression and satisfaction with care, but they did not find a positive impact on HbA1c[51] or on self-care, as measured by healthy nutrition, physical activity, or smoking cessation.[65] A subsequent analysis revealed that the greatest impact on reducing depressive symptoms was experienced by patients with the highest severity of medical problems (2 or more complications).[66] A similar study (the Improving Mood-Promoting Access to Collaborative [IMPACT] trial, also using a depression care manager) reported a very large increase in depression-free days (approximately 115 more over a 24-month period) and a balancing of increased mental health costs by nearly equal reductions in medical services.[67] This study did not examine effects on glycemic control, but similar findings (i.e., good benefit for depression treatment insofar as the depression itself is concerned, but no measurable impact on diabetes-specific outcomes) were reported elsewhere.[53] In other antidepressant treatment findings, a recent study (n = 152) reported prolonged depression-free intervals from maintenance therapy with sertraline following recovery from major depression, along with improvements in HgbA1c levels for at least 1 year,[68] while another, much smaller study (n = 15) reported a beneficial effect on insulin sensitivity from treatment with paroxetine.[69]

A study reporting benefits for both depression and diabetes as a result of depression treatment assessed the efficacy of cognitive-behavioral therapy (CBT). This study, published in 1998, reported the following outcomes: "CBT combined with diabetes education is an effective nonpharmacological treatment for major depression in patients with diabetes.... This therapy was associated with improvement in glycemic control despite its association with a decline in self-monitoring of blood glucose levels."[52] However, a more recent study did not replicate these findings.[70]

In summary, it is difficult at this stage of the research to draw any firm conclusions about the likelihood of improvement in glycemic control that may emanate from successful treatment of depression; however, it does seem clear that treating depression in diabetics will improve depressive symptoms, and it seems possible that certain treatments may also have beneficial effects on glycemic control. Until we have studies that carefully differentiate partial from full responders to depression treatment, we won't know what the real potential for improving glycemic control through treating depression might be.

Depression, heart disease, hypertension, and stroke — Due to the metabolic interconnections between cardiovascular and cerebrovascular conditions, a separate analysis of the two as they relate to depression is beyond the scope of this monograph. Underlying mechanisms connect many of the effects and outcomes,[71] and it is possible that the increased risk contributed by depression to the mortality and morbidity of these conditions is primarily connected to those underlying mechanisms, rather than being correlated directly to the diagnostic entities themselves. Possible mechanisms that may link depression, heart disease, hypertension, and stroke include hyperactivity of the HPA and sympathetic-adrenal-medullary (SAM) systems, diminished heart rate variability, and platelet activation and inflammation.[8, 71] Some of these processes will be examined further in Chapter 6; here, we simply acknowledge the principle of functional medicine that indicates that *disturbances in underlying common metabolic pathways contribute to diverse phenotypic expression* (i.e., different diseases).

As with diabetes, important information has recently emerged indicating that it is the depression that most often precedes the coronary event, rather than the reverse.[72] It is also becoming apparent that stroke is the specific cardio/cerebrovascular element with which depressive symptoms are most strongly associated, rather than myocardial infarction (MI), coronary artery disease (CAD), or heart failure.[15, 73] Multiple studies emphasize that depression is an independent risk factor for stroke, even after controlling for a very large array of variables.[74-76] The risk of stroke increases as the number of depressive symptoms rises, indicating the lack of a single decisive threshold for concern.[77]

Although the research on the link between depression and hypertension is not nearly as definitive as that for heart disease and stroke, there are many studies documenting an association with depressive symptoms[76, 78-82] and decreased compliance with antihypertensive regimens for patients with comorbid depression.[83, 84] The many interconnections between depression, heart disease, hypertension, and stroke are multidirectional. For example, we know that risk factors for stroke include hypertension, heart disease, and depression; risk factors for cardiovascular disease include hypertension and depression; risk factors for hypertension include many of the same psychosocial and behavioral elements that contribute to depression and heart disease; and risk factors for depression include all 3 conditions—heart disease, hypertension, and stroke. Isolating each condition and treating it independently simply does not reflect the very real and powerful (web-like) mechanisms at work in each person.

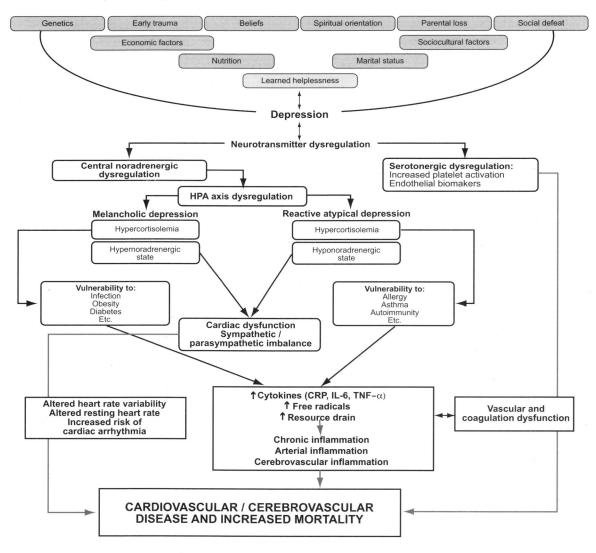

Figure 3.1—The Depression-Cardiovascular Disease Connection

Many studies have documented associations between depression and CAD,[85-88] MI,[86, 89, 90] and heart failure.[91, 92] Mortality is much higher for cardiac patients with depression (both mortality from all causes and cardiac death)[85, 89, 90] and for stroke patients with depression.[73, 76] These associations remain significant even more than 10 years after hospitalization, and the severity of the depression correlates strongly with increased risk.[85] A 1996 study reported that "patients with moderate to severe depression had a 69% greater odds of cardiac death and a 78% greater odds of mortality from all causes than nondepressed patients."[85] A decade later, a lengthy analysis of the evidence published in 2005 by the Agency for Healthcare Research and Quality indicated that "depression appears to be associated with about a 3-fold increased risk of cardiac mortality."[90]

Depression increases the risk for the onset of coronary disease in healthy people, both etiologically and prognostically.[86-88, 93] As an independent risk factor, depression confers a risk greater than that related to smoking.[93] As mentioned briefly above, many hypotheses about the mechanisms of this relationship have been discussed. The most compelling were summarized in a review by Joynt[94]:

- Dysregulation of the HPA axis, documented consistently in patients with depression, can also exacerbate the development of cardiovascular disease. HPA hyperactivity heightens sympathoadrenal hyperactivity (fight/flight), which can increase plasma catecholamines, leading to vasoconstriction, platelet activation, and elevated heart rate, all damaging to the cardiovascular system when present over extended periods of time (as in depressive episodes).
- Rhythm disturbances are found in cardiac patients with a poor prognosis and have been noted in patients with depression.
- A heightened inflammatory state has been well documented in both heart disease and depression. This may be a downstream result of a primary process such as HPA axis dysregulation, or it may arise from chronic infection elsewhere in the body (e.g., periodontal disease, chronic viral disease, gastrointestinal inflammatory disease); however, we cannot yet say whether inflammation is a contributing cause of depression or whether depression itself causes inflammation. It is possible that the process is web-like (multidirectional), as are so many other biological processes.
- Hypercoagulability is associated with both the development and prognosis for heart disease, and evidence of hypercoagulability has been found in studies of depressed patients.

Does treating the depression improve markers of heart disease? At least 2 major studies have investigated that question.[95, 96] While beneficial effects on depression were found in both studies (consistent with effects on noncardiac patients with depression), no effects on measures of heart disease were reported. A more recent study investigating only the effect on depression in post-MI or post-revascularization patients (or those with coronary angiography showing 50% or more blockage in at least one major coronary artery) supported an effect size of 31% over placebo for the use of citalopram administered in conjunction with weekly clinical management sessions for patients with both CAD and depression (measured by change between baseline and 12 weeks on the Hamilton Depression Rating Scale).[97] The benefits were greater for patients with recurring depression, rather than those with first episodes. (This same study did not show an effect of interpersonal psychotherapy.) A positive effect on mortality and reinfarction (event-free survival) was noted for post-MI patients treated with selective serotonin reuptake inhibitors (SSRIs) in a large observational secondary analysis of the Enhancing Recovery in Coronary Heart Disease (ENRICHD) study.[98] Animal studies have documented antiplatelet effects of sertraline and N-desmethylsertraline, which may explain the mortality benefits of SSRIs after ischemic events.[99]

It is important to remember, however, that these results are for patients *who have been treated for depression but are not necessarily in full recovery*. As mentioned above, we know that full and lasting remission is found in only about one third of treated patients. Furthermore, we don't know how long it might take after full recovery for the effects of chronic depression, which may have accumulated over many years, to subside and allow underlying mechanisms to return to a healthier state. We hope that future research will evaluate these issues more fully.

To summarize, the impact of depression on the course of an extensive array of chronic diseases is well documented in the literature. The preceding detailed discussions of the depression-diabetes and depression-cardio/cerebrovascular relationships have identified some common underlying themes that also surface in reports of many other chronic diseases and their relationship to depression, particularly:

- The temporal primacy of depression in comorbid conditions
- The much greater risk of poor outcomes when depression occurs in the presence of a significant chronic disease
- The need for improved screening and treatment
- The multidirectional nature of the relationships

The question of demonstrating improved medical outcomes as a result of treating the comorbid depression in chronic disease is addressed in a recent article by Katon, wherein he discussed 2 chronic disease treatment studies showing that "improvement in depression outcome was associated with decreased somatic symptoms *without improvement in physiological measures* [italics added]."[100] In other words, perhaps quality of life improves although disease markers do not, or perhaps treatment alone does not have the desired effect because the disease is still present for two thirds of those treated. We need long-term studies on patients whose depression goes into full and long-lasting remission before we will know whether we can also reverse physiological disease markers by treating comorbid depression.

We will highlight a few other common disease-depression relationships below to further emphasize the critical importance of improving assessment and treatment of depression in clinical practice.

Depression and asthma/allergy — Both allergy and asthma have been associated with depression. A study of 1094 patients with allergy, anxiety, or PMS revealed that 21% of allergy patients had a recurrent problem with brief depression; of those, half reported at least moderately severe symptoms. None were being treated for depression (a diagnosis of depression was an exclusion criterion).[101] Another study comparing the effects of depression and anxiety on asthma determined that both conditions were responsible for reduced quality of life, but only depressive disorders were associated with worse asthma control.[102] A sizable study of 767 youth with asthma identified 125 (16.2%) with one or more anxiety or depressive disorders; that subgroup reported significantly more days with asthma symptoms than the subjects with no anxiety or depressive disorders, and the overall number of reported asthma symptoms was significantly associated with the number of anxiety and depressive symptoms.[103] A prospective cohort of 743 adults with asthma (recruited after a hospitalization for asthma) showed a prevalence of depressive symptoms of 18%.[104]

These studies and many others[102, 105-108] are consistent in demonstrating that the presence of depression in those with asthma significantly reduces both treatment success and quality of life indicators. Although we did not find any clinical trials studying the impact on asthma outcomes of providing screening and treatment for depression, depressed asthma patients will continue to experience worse disease outcomes than nondepressed asthma patients, resulting in considerable unnecessary suffering and reduced quality of life. Practitioners must be cognizant of "the potential risk of poorer asthma control and functional impairment in this population."[107]

Depression and autoimmunity — Patients with autoimmune conditions such as rheumatoid arthritis[27, 109, 110] and systemic lupus erythematosus[111, 112] report higher levels of depression, and often the depression goes untreated as the clinician focuses on management of the primary diagnosis. The consequences of untreated depression in these conditions are increased mortality[27] (including a suicide risk[112]) and poorer treatment outcomes.[100, 113]

Depression in patients with multiple sclerosis has been reported at much higher rates than in the general population, correlating primarily with severity of disease but also with younger age, lower education, and lack of social support.[114] Attempts to localize the depressive symptoms to certain areas of the brain have not produced any consistent findings, but a 2005 review of imaging studies indicated that "the evidence seems to favour an association between depression in multiple sclerosis with greater neuropathology in the left anterior temporal/parietal regions."[115] The most disturbing evidence reported by these reviewers is that among multiple sclerosis patients with major depression, two thirds were "not receiving antidepressants and a third of suicidal patients had not received any psychological assistance." Perhaps this is one of the reasons that suicide rates in multiple sclerosis patients are very high.[116, 117]

Although it is true that depression and medical conditions can have many shared symptoms and that there are common pathways to both (such as HPA axis disturbances and changes in immunologic function[118, 119]), there appears to be an alarming failure on the part of physicians to screen for—and then treat—the depression that is so very common in multiple sclerosis[120] (and other chronic diseases).

An association between autoimmune thyroiditis and depression has been reported; although a recent article reported that "depression is not characterized by an overt thyroid dysfunction... a subgroup of depressed patients may manifest subtle thyroid abnormalities, or an activation of an autoimmune process."[121] One article hypothesized that "the psychiatric disorders and the autoimmune reaction seem to be rooted in a same (and not easily correctable) aberrancy in the immuno-endocrine system."[122] Another study suggested that autoimmune abnormalities in neurotransmitter receptors might be associated with psychiatric symptoms.[123] These hypotheses concerning cause have yet to be proved, but the connection between autoimmunity and depression is clear enough that clinicians treating patients with autoimmune conditions should also screen for and treat depression.

Depression and cancer — A cancer diagnosis increases psychosocial stress on many levels—fears of dying, disability, treatment side effects, pain, and economic distress can all contribute to a natural sadness response. A relevant question is whether chronic stress, with the resulting increase in allostatic load, is a factor in the association of depression with cancer.[124] A significant challenge in researching depression among cancer patients has been to distinguish clearly between a depressive disorder and the symptoms of an appropriate but usually temporary response to bad news.[125] An additional challenge has been determining the effect on cancer outcomes of depressive disorders, given the similarity of many depressive symptoms to those experienced during cancer treatment (fatigue, weight loss, sleep disturbance, decreased libido, anorexia, etc.).[126]

Interestingly, most cancer patients do not experience a major depression.[126] Researchers are working to identify and study the factors that affect the prevalence of depression in cancer patients, which has been estimated at anywhere from 8 to 33%.[127] Reasons for the great variation in findings are many, including the stage at diagnosis, treatment prognosis, length of and debility associated with treatment, and the fact that stage at diagnosis was not always taken into account in the various studies.[125, 127] Unfortunately, there is no standard approach to diagnosing depression in cancer patients, so it is difficult to extract comparable information from the many studies; a validated screening instrument that distinguishes between common symptoms of cancer and cancer treatment and those of depression is needed. Nonetheless, there is widespread acknowledgment of a high prevalence of depressive symptoms among various types of cancers.[126, 128, 129] Sadly, there is evidence to indicate that "up to 80% of the psychological and psychiatric morbidity which develops in cancer patients goes unrecognized and untreated."[125]

In a 2007 review, Pasquini and Biondi[127] reported that the consequences of untreated depression in cancer patients are reduced quality of life, reduced compliance with treatment, and prolonged hospitalization. In addition, they noted that "psychological status seems to predict the length of survival in several types of cancer such as melanoma, non-small-cell lung cancer, breast and kidney cancer." Groenvald et al[130] also reported that low levels of psychological distress independently predicted longer recurrence-free and overall survival, after controlling for biological factors. Even for dying patients, proper treatment for depression can prevent or alleviate a greatly diminished quality of life.[131]

In 1998, Holden et al[132] proposed "a causal model in which the relationship between stress, depression and carcinoma is clarified." This model proposes that stress and depression foster tumor progression via inhibition of the expression of surface cell major histocompatibility (MHC) class I and II molecules, altered cytokine expression, and reduced natural killer cell activity. While consistent with the concept of systems biology and interconnectivity and the depression-osteoporosis link discussed below, much research needs to be done to prove this model is active in humans with depression.

Depression and osteoporosis — Approximately 10 million Americans have osteoporosis and 34 million Americans are at risk for it, making it a major public health issue.[133] The association between osteoporosis and depression first emerged in the research literature in the 1980s. The evidence of this association over the past 25 years has been consistently strong (although not unanimous), with some studies detecting decreased bone mineral density[134-136] and others identifying increased risk for fractures[137 138, 139] in both men and women of various ethnicities.

Initially, the common assumption of researchers was that the pain, deformity, and increasing fragility of osteoporosis caused sufficient stress to create reactive depression in many patients.[140]

However, the perspective on causality has evolved considerably. More recent and more carefully structured investigations have revealed a complex relationship between the 2 conditions that is almost certainly bidirectional, but with depression primarily influencing the development of osteoporosis, rather than the reverse.[134] Because depression is often common at younger ages than osteoporosis, longitudinal studies have been able to observe what happens to bone maintenance in depressed patients over time. Depression has, indeed, emerged as a significant risk factor for men (studies show some surprising levels of risk[135, 141]) and both pre- and postmenopausal women.[137, 142-144] Why?

The strongest hypothesis at this time is that the hypercortisolism and associated immune and endocrine dysfunctions frequently seen in typical depression affect bone loss,[142, 144] with the effects sometimes detectable even in the very early stages of depressive illness.[143] In the functional medicine model, depression can be said to have multiple roles in the development of osteoporosis, functioning as antecedent, trigger, and mediator. Although it would be premature to say that the scientific consensus is now definitive, there is some very persuasive evidence that these well-known endocrine/inflammatory dysfunctions are powerful contributing factors for the risk of osteoporosis.[136, 142, 144] A model of this process is described in a 2006 review of depression and osteoporosis in men[141]: "A potential mechanism of bone loss in depression has been proposed, involving concurrent activation of the HPA and sympatho-adrenal axes, suppression of the gonadal and somatotrophic axes, and high interleukin-6 and low leptin levels." Figure 3.2 provides a graphic representation of this model.

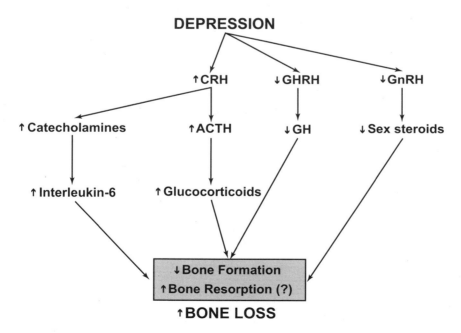

Figure 3.2—Bone Loss in Depression
Source: Ilias I, et al. *Hormones*. 2006;5(1):9-16.

We can see here the endocrine and immune effects of chronic HPA axis hyperactivity (most clearly present in pure melancholic depressives rather than atypical, reactive depressives), and we can also begin to draw some important conclusions about common pathways linking the development of many chronic conditions that have been associated with depression: heart disease, diabetes, stroke, and osteoporosis, but probably others as well. That is not to say that the single underlying cause has been found. A 2005 study of depressed patients identified elevations in plasma interleukin-6 even in the absence of hypercortisolism,[145] indicating that there may be other inflammatory mechanisms at work. However, the HPA axis model that is clearly part of depressive illness appears to be a significant mediating factor for depressive disorders, as well as many comorbid conditions; untreated HPA axis dysregulation may also contribute to the difficulty of treating these medical conditions effectively, unless the depression and its chronic effects can be resolved. The implications for both prevention and treatment are profound.

Depression and obesity — Obesity may be the fastest growing chronic disease in the world. The *New England Journal of Medicine* reported in 2007 that "more than 1.1 billion adults worldwide are overweight, and 312 million of them are obese. In addition, at least 155 million children worldwide are overweight or obese."[146] Because obesity is a powerful driver for the development of diabetes and heart disease,[147] this creates a public health challenge of almost unimaginable magnitude. It is fueled by cultural and environmental changes that are difficult, if not impossible, to arrest or reverse. Sedentary lives, fragmented communities, easy access to calorie-heavy but nutrition-deficient foods, and high levels of psychological stress are all elements of this complex situation.[148]

As with many of the conditions we have discussed, early research on the association of depression and obesity often returned conflicting results, with some studies reporting an association and others not finding it.[147, 149] Methodological issues such as failure to standardize the definition of depression, failure to standardize the criteria and limits for levels of obesity, the diversity in age and physical health of participants, and the use of community versus clinic- or hospital-based samples have all been cited as factors in the divergence of early reports.[147, 149] Investigations that have attempted to control for the earlier methodological problems have found more consistent results, which could be summarized (with some loss of specificity) in the following way:

- Severe/morbid obesity is strongly associated with depression for both men and women.[150-156]
- Mild obesity is also associated, although less strongly, with depression in women.[147, 153]
- Mild obesity is inversely associated with depression in men.[147]
- The associations between obesity and depression are stronger in the presence of other illnesses.[156]
- The positive effects are more pronounced when clinic- or hospital-based populations are studied.[157]
- Although metabolic syndrome is not always associated with obesity, it very often is; nondepressed women and men with metabolic syndrome are twice as likely to develop depressive symptoms later in their lives.[58]

Findings in children are not markedly different. Depression is most strongly associated with higher levels of obesity, although in children, and to some degree in adults, it is harder to detect whether depression causes obesity or obesity causes depression.[158] As with other conditions discussed above, the relationship appears to be bidirectional, with obesity influencing the development of depression and depression affecting the prevalence of obesity,[156] but there is not as yet a clear picture of which directionality might be the stronger.

Common mechanisms underlying both of these debilitating conditions have become apparent, representing dysfunctions that are a result of a growing mismatch between genes and environment that threatens to engulf all the world's communities. An interesting mechanism study in 2005 identified visceral adipose tissue (VAT), as differentiated from subcutaneous adipose tissue (SAT), as the particular type of fat that is associated with depression. Increased interleukin-6 is said to result from increased visceral adiposity, which perhaps points to some of the inflammatory mechanisms at work.[150] A compelling presentation of hypercortisolism and the disturbed HPA axis (resulting in increased interleukin-6, as described above under *Depression and osteoporosis*) as the common underlying mechanisms was made by Bornstein et al in 2006,[159] who stated, "Altogether, there is unequivocal evidence for a key role of the HPA axis in both obesity and depression…. Shared biology does not mean identical or uniform mechanisms of disease, but rather systems that interact, sometimes augmenting one another, and at other times canceling each other out." Other studies[160, 161] have linked endotoxemia to obesity and insulin resistance, as well as to changes in mood.

Once again, we are drawn to the inescapable conclusion that despite myriad variations in presentations and diagnoses, there are nonetheless some common, identifiable antecedents, triggers, and mediators of many of the world's most common, costly, and debilitating chronic diseases. As the evidence base emerges and strengthens, and the role of depression in both prevalence and outcomes grows clearer, these facts should redirect our attention away from treating disease-specific symptoms and toward remediating underlying dysfunctions, whether those dysfunctions are at the societal or the individual level. We have a surfeit of factual information about the physiological and biochemical factors at work in depression and those conditions with which it is comorbid, most of which has not been translated, as of this date, into the treatment model for depression. As we proceed through this monograph, we will bring together the environmental, cultural, and psychosocial factors that drive our biochemistry and physiology toward dysfunction, and we will present an integrated and more comprehensive approach to treatment.

References

1. Sullivan PF, Neale MC, Kendler KS. Genetic epidemiology of major depression: review and meta-analysis. *Am J Psychiatry*. 2000;157:1552-1562.
2. Hasin DS, Goodwin RD, Stinson FS, Grant BF. Epidemiology of major depressive disorder: results from the National Epidemiologic Survey on Alcoholism and Related Conditions. *Arch Gen Psychiatry*. 2005;62:1097-1106.
3. Kessler RC, Berglund P, Demler O, et al. The epidemiology of major depressive disorder: results from the National Comorbidity Survey Replication (NCS-R). *JAMA*. 2003;289:3095-3105.
4. Bourdon KH, Rae DS, Locke BZ, Narrow WE, Regier DA. Estimating the prevalence of mental disorders in U.S. adults from the Epidemiologic Catchment Area Survey. *Public Health Rep*. 1992;107:663-668.
5. Kessler RC, Nelson CB, McGonagle KA, Liu J, Swartz M, Blazer DG. Comorbidity of DSM-III-R major depressive disorder in the general population: results from the US National Comorbidity Survey. *Br J Psychiatry Suppl*. 1996:17-30.
6. *Diagnostic and Statistical Manual of Mental Disorders, Fourth Edition, Text Revision (DSM-IV-TR)*. Arlington, VA: American Psychiatric Association; 2000.
7. Kessler RC, Berglund P, Demler O, Jin R, Merikangas KR, Walters EE. Lifetime prevalence and age-of-onset distributions of DSM-IV disorders in the National Comorbidity Survey Replication. *Arch Gen Psychiatry*. 2005;62:593-602.
8. Kopp MS, Rethelyi J. Where psychology meets physiology: chronic stress and premature mortality--the Central-Eastern European health paradox. *Brain Res Bull*. 2004;62:351-367.
9. Noble RE. Depression in women. *Metabolism*. 2005;54:49-52.
10. Burt VK, Stein K. Epidemiology of depression throughout the female life cycle. *J Clin Psychiatry*. 2002;63 Suppl 7:9-15.
11. Schmidt PJ, Haq N, Rubinow DR. A longitudinal evaluation of the relationship between reproductive status and mood in perimenopausal women. *Am J Psychiatry*. 2004;161:2238-2244.
12. Cohen LS, Soares CN, Vitonis AF, Otto MW, Harlow BL. Risk for new onset of depression during the menopausal transition: the Harvard study of moods and cycles. *Arch Gen Psychiatry*. 2006;63:385-390.
13. Rasgon NL, Altshuler LL, Fairbanks LA, et al. Estrogen replacement therapy in the treatment of major depressive disorder in perimenopausal women. *J Clin Psychiatry*. 2002;63 Suppl 7:45-48.
14. Douma SL, Husband C, O'Donnell ME, Barwin BN, Woodend AK. Estrogen-related mood disorders: reproductive life cycle factors. *ANS Adv Nurs Sci*. 2005;28:364-375.
15. Salaycik KJ, Kelly-Hayes M, Beiser A, et al. Depressive symptoms and risk of stroke: the Framingham Study. *Stroke*. 2007;38:16-21.
16. Kendler KS, Gardner CO, Gatz M, Pedersen NL. The sources of co-morbidity between major depression and generalized anxiety disorder in a Swedish national twin sample. *Psychol Med*. 2007;37:453-462.
17. Kessing LV. Epidemiology of subtypes of depression. *Acta Psychiatr Scand Suppl*. 2007:85-89.
18. Turner RJ, Lloyd DA. Stress burden and the lifetime incidence of psychiatric disorder in young adults: racial and ethnic contrasts. *Arch Gen Psychiatry*. 2004;61:481-488.
19. Schreiber R. Wandering in the dark: women's experiences with depression. *Health Care Women Int*. 2001;22:85-98.
20. Ge X, Natsuaki MN, Conger RD. Trajectories of depressive symptoms and stressful life events among male and female adolescents in divorced and nondivorced families. *Dev Psychopathol*. 2006;18:253-273.
21. Huurre T, Junkkari H, Aro H. Long-term psychosocial effects of parental divorce: a follow-up study from adolescence to adulthood. *Eur Arch Psychiatry Clin Neurosci*. 2006;256:256-263.
22. Schulz R, Beach SR, Ives DG, Martire LM, Ariyo AA, Kop WJ. Association between depression and mortality in older adults: the Cardiovascular Health Study. *Arch Intern Med*. 2000;160:1761-1768.
23. Wilson RS, Bienias JL, Mendes de Leon CF, Evans DA, Bennett DA. Negative affect and mortality in older persons. *Am J Epidemiol*. 2003;158:827-835.
24. Goldacre MJ, Duncan ME, Griffith M, Cook-Mozaffari P. Psychiatric disorders certified on death certificates in an English population. *Soc Psychiatry Psychiatr Epidemiol*. 2006;41:409-414.
25. Adamson JA, Price GM, Breeze E, Bulpitt CJ, Fletcher AE. Are older people dying of depression? Findings from the Medical Research Council trial of the assessment and management of older people in the community. *J Am Geriatr Soc*. 2005;53:1128-1132.
26. Everson-Rose SA, House JS, Mero RP. Depressive symptoms and mortality risk in a national sample: confounding effects of health status. *Psychosom Med*. 2004;66:823-830.

27. Ang DC, Choi H, Kroenke K, Wolfe F. Comorbid depression is an independent risk factor for mortality in patients with rheumatoid arthritis. *J Rheumatol.* 2005;32:1013-1019.

28. Whooley MA, Browner WS. Association between depressive symptoms and mortality in older women. Study of Osteoporotic Fractures Research Group. *Arch Intern Med.* 1998;158:2129-2135.

29. Angst J, Angst F, Gerber-Werder R, Gamma A. Suicide in 406 mood-disorder patients with and without long-term medication: a 40 to 44 years' follow-up. *Arch Suicide Res.* 2005;9:279-300.

30. Lecrubier Y. Widespread underrecognition and undertreatment of anxiety and mood disorders: results from 3 European studies. *J Clin Psychiatry.* 2007;68 Suppl 2:36-41.

31. Anderson GF, Chu E. Expanding priorities--Confronting chronic disease in countries with low income. *N Engl J Med.* 2007;356:209-211.

32. McCollum M, Ellis SL, Regensteiner JG, Zhang W, Sullivan PW. Minor depression and health status among US adults with diabetes mellitus. *Am J Manag Care.* 2007;13:65-72.

33. WHO Initiative on Depression in Public Health. http://www.who.int/mental_health/management/depression/depressioninph/en/. Accessed March 10, 2008.

34. Palpant RG, Steimnitz R, Bornemann TH, Hawkins K. The Carter Center Mental Health Program: Addressing the public health crisis in the field of mental health through policy change and stigma reduction. *Preventing Chronic Disease.* 2006;3:1-6.

35. Mikolajczyk RT, Bredehorst M, Khelaifat N, Maier C, Maxwell AE. Correlates of depressive symptoms among Latino and Non-Latino white adolescents: Findings from the 2003 California Health Interview Survey. *BMC Public Health.* 2007;21.

36. Mykletun A, Overland S, Dahl AA, et al. A population-based cohort study of the effect of common mental disorders on disability pension awards. *Am J Psychiatry.* 2006;163:1412-1418.

37. Stewart WF, Ricci JA, Chee E, Hahn SR, Morganstein D. Cost of lost productive work time among US workers with depression. *JAMA.* 2003;289:3135-3144.

38. Adler DA, McLaughlin TJ, Rogers WH, Chang H, Lapitsky L, Lerner D. Job performance deficits due to depression. *Am J Psychiatry.* 2006;163:1569-1576.

39. Olshansky SJ, Passaro DJ, Hershow RC, et al. A potential decline in life expectancy in the United States in the 21st century. *N Engl J Med.* 2005;352:1138-1145.

40. Chapman DP, Perry GS, Strine TW. The vital link between chronic disease and depressive disorders. *Preventing Chronic Disease.* 2005;2:1-10.

41. Langa KM, Valenstein MA, Fendrick AM, Kabeto MU, Vijan S. Extent and cost of informal caregiving for older Americans with symptoms of depression. *Am J Psychiatry.* 2004;161:857-863.

42. Kessler RC, McGonagle KA, Zhao S, et al. Lifetime and 12-month prevalence of DSM-III-R psychiatric disorders in the United States. Results from the National Comorbidity Survey. *Arch Gen Psychiatry.* 1994;51:8-19.

43. Keles H, Ekici A, Ekici M, Bulcun E, Altinkaya V. Effect of chronic diseases and associated psychological distress on health-related quality of life. *Intern Med J.* 2007;37:6-11.

44. Stahl SM. Why settle for silver, when you can go for gold? Response vs. recovery as the goal of antidepressant therapy. *J Clin Psychiatry.* 1999;60:213-214.

45. Hanninen JA, Takala JK, Keinanen-Kiukaanniemi SM. Depression in subjects with type 2 diabetes. Predictive factors and relation to quality of life. *Diabetes Care.* 1999;22:997-998.

46. Egede LE, Nietert PJ, Zheng D. Depression and all-cause and coronary heart disease mortality among adults with and without diabetes. *Diabetes Care.* 2005;28:1339-1345.

47. Rubin RR, Ciechanowski P, Egede LE, Lin EH, Lustman PJ. Recognizing and treating depression in patients with diabetes. *Curr Diab Rep.* 2004;4:119-125.

48. Anderson RJ, Freedland KE, Clouse RE, Lustman PJ. The prevalence of comorbid depression in adults with diabetes: a meta-analysis. *Diabetes Care.* 2001;24:1069-1078.

49. Zhang X, Norris SL, Gregg EW, Cheng YJ, Beckles G, Kahn HS. Depressive symptoms and mortality among persons with and without diabetes. *Am J Epidemiol.* 2005;161:652-660.

50. Ciechanowski PS, Katon WJ, Russo JE. Depression and diabetes: impact of depressive symptoms on adherence, function, and costs. *Arch Intern Med.* 2000;160:3278-3285.

51. Katon WJ, Von Korff M, Lin EH, et al. The Pathways Study: a randomized trial of collaborative care in patients with diabetes and depression. *Arch Gen Psychiatry.* 2004;61:1042-1049.

52. Lustman PJ, Griffith LS, Freedland KE, Kissel SS, Clouse RE. Cognitive behavior therapy for depression in type 2 diabetes mellitus. A randomized, controlled trial. *Ann Intern Med.* 1998;129:613-621.

53. Williams JW, Jr., Katon W, Lin EH, et al. The effectiveness of depression care management on diabetes-related outcomes in older patients. *Ann Intern Med.* 2004;140:1015-1024.

54. Olsson I, Mykletun A, Dahl AA. General practitioners' self-perceived ability to recognize severity of common mental disorders: an underestimated factor in case identification? *Clin Pract Epidemol Ment Health.* 2006;2:21.

55. Lustman PJ, Williams MM, Sayuk GS, Nix BD, Clouse RE. Factors influencing glycemic control in type 2 diabetes during acute- and maintenance-phase treatment of major depressive disorder with bupropion. *Diabetes Care.* 2007;30:459-466.

56. Talbot F, Nouwen A. A review of the relationship between depression and diabetes in adults: is there a link? *Diabetes Care.* 2000;23:1556-1562.

57. Katon W, Von Korff M, Lin E, et al. Improving primary care treatment of depression among patients with diabetes mellitus: the design of the pathways study. *Gen Hosp Psychiatry.* 2003;25:158-168.

58. Koponen H, Jokelainen J, Keinanen-Kiukaanniemi S, Kumpusalo E, Vanhala M. Metabolic Syndrome Predisposes to Depressive Symptoms: A Population-Based 7-Year Follow-Up Study. *J Clin Psychiatry.* 2008:e1-e5.

59. Lustman PJ, Anderson RJ, Freedland KE, de Groot M, Carney RM, Clouse RE. Depression and poor glycemic control: a meta-analytic review of the literature. *Diabetes Care.* 2000;23:934-942.

60. de Groot M, Jacobson AM, Samson JA, Welch G. Glycemic control and major depression in patients with type 1 and type 2 diabetes mellitus. *J Psychosom Res.* 1999;46:425-435.

61. Van Tilburg MA, McCaskill CC, Lane JD, et al. Depressed mood is a factor in glycemic control in type 1 diabetes. *Psychosom Med.* 2001;63:551-555.

62. Musselman DL, Betan E, Larsen H, Phillips LS. Relationship of depression to diabetes types 1 and 2: epidemiology, biology, and treatment. *Biol Psychiatry*. 2003;54:317-329.

63. Lustman PJ, Freedland KE, Griffith LS, Clouse RE. Fluoxetine for depression in diabetes: a randomized double-blind placebo-controlled trial. *Diabetes Care*. 2000;23:618-623.

64. Lustman PJ, Griffith LS, Clouse RE, et al. Effects of nortriptyline on depression and glycemic control in diabetes: results of a double-blind, placebo-controlled trial. *Psychosom Med*. 1997;59:241-250.

65. Lin EH, Katon W, Rutter C, et al. Effects of enhanced depression treatment on diabetes self-care. *Ann Fam Med*. 2006;4:46-53.

66. Kinder LS, Katon WJ, Ludman E, et al. Improving depression care in patients with diabetes and multiple complications. *J Gen Intern Med*. 2006;21:1036-1041.

67. Katon W, Unutzer J, Fan MY, et al. Cost-effectiveness and net benefit of enhanced treatment of depression for older adults with diabetes and depression. *Diabetes Care*. 2006;29:265-270.

68. Lustman PJ, Clouse RE, Nix BD, et al. Sertraline for prevention of depression recurrence in diabetes mellitus: a randomized, double-blind, placebo-controlled trial. *Arch Gen Psychiatry*. 2006;63:521-529.

69. Paile-Hyvarinen M, Wahlbeck K, Eriksson JG. Quality of life and metabolic status in mildly depressed women with type 2 diabetes treated with paroxetine: a single-blind randomised placebo controlled trial. *BMC Fam Pract*. 2003;4:7.

70. van der Ven NC, Hogenelst MH, Tromp-Wever AM, et al. Short-term effects of cognitive behavioural group training (CBGT) in adult Type 1 diabetes patients in prolonged poor glycaemic control. A randomized controlled trial. *Diabet Med*. 2005;22:1619-1623.

71. Carod-Artal FJ. Are mood disorders a stroke risk factor? *Stroke*. 2007;38:1-3.

72. Glassman AH, Bigger JT, Jr. Antidepressants in coronary heart disease: SSRIs reduce depression, but do they save lives? *JAMA*. 2007;297:411-412.

73. Gump BB, Matthews KA, Eberly LE, Chang YF. Depressive symptoms and mortality in men: results from the Multiple Risk Factor Intervention Trial. *Stroke*. 2005;36:98-102.

74. Jonas BS, Mussolino ME. Symptoms of depression as a prospective risk factor for stroke. *Psychosom Med*. 2000;62:463-471.

75. Ohira T, Iso H, Satoh S, et al. Prospective study of depressive symptoms and risk of stroke among japanese. *Stroke*. 2001;32:903-908.

76. Everson SA, Roberts RE, Goldberg DE, Kaplan GA. Depressive symptoms and increased risk of stroke mortality over a 29-year period. *Arch Intern Med*. 1998;158:1133-1138.

77. Ostir GV, Markides KS, Peek MK, Goodwin JS. The association between emotional well-being and the incidence of stroke in older adults. *Psychosom Med*. 2001;63:210-215.

78. Jonas BS, Lando JF. Negative affect as a prospective risk factor for hypertension. *Psychosom Med*. 2000;62:188-196.

79. Scherrer JF, Xian H, Bucholz KK, et al. A twin study of depression symptoms, hypertension, and heart disease in middle-aged men. *Psychosom Med*. 2003;65:548-557.

80. Rutledge T, Hogan BE. A quantitative review of prospective evidence linking psychological factors with hypertension development. *Psychosom Med*. 2002;64:758-766.

81. Meyer CM, Armenian HK, Eaton WW, Ford DE. Incident hypertension associated with depression in the Baltimore Epidemiologic Catchment area follow-up study. *J Affect Disord*. 2004;83:127-133.

82. Davidson K, Jonas BS, Dixon KE, Markovitz JH. Do depression symptoms predict early hypertension incidence in young adults in the CARDIA study? Coronary Artery Risk Development in Young Adults. *Arch Intern Med*. 2000;160:1495-1500.

83. Wang PS, Avorn J, Brookhart MA, et al. Effects of noncardiovascular comorbidities on antihypertensive use in elderly hypertensives. *Hypertension*. 2005;46:273-279.

84. Morris AB, Li J, Kroenke K, Bruner-England TE, Young JM, Murray MD. Factors associated with drug adherence and blood pressure control in patients with hypertension. *Pharmacotherapy*. 2006;26:483-492.

85. Barefoot JC, Helms MJ, Mark DB, et al. Depression and long-term mortality risk in patients with coronary artery disease. *Am J Cardiol*. 1996;78:613-617.

86. Rugulies R. Depression as a predictor for coronary heart disease. a review and meta-analysis. *Am J Prev Med*. 2002;23:51-61.

87. Wulsin LR. Is depression a major risk factor for coronary disease? A systematic review of the epidemiologic evidence. *Harv Rev Psychiatry*. 2004;12:79-93.

88. Frasure-Smith N, Lesperance F. Recent evidence linking coronary heart disease and depression. *Can J Psychiatry*. 2006;51:730-737.

89. Barefoot JC, Schroll M. Symptoms of depression, acute myocardial infarction, and total mortality in a community sample. *Circulation*. 1996;93:1976-1980.

90. Bush DE, Ziegelstein RC, Patel UV, et al. Post-myocardial infarction depression. *Evid Rep Technol Assess (Summ)*. 2005:1-8.

91. Sherwood A, Blumenthal JA, Trivedi R, et al. Relationship of depression to death or hospitalization in patients with heart failure. *Arch Intern Med*. 2007;167:367-373.

92. Johansson P, Dahlstrom U, Brostrom A. Consequences and predictors of depression in patients with chronic heart failure: implications for nursing care and future research. *Prog Cardiovasc Nurs*. 2006;21:202-211.

93. Wulsin LR, Singal BM. Do depressive symptoms increase the risk for the onset of coronary disease? A systematic quantitative review. *Psychosom Med*. 2003;65:201-210.

94. Joynt KE, Whellan DJ, O'Connor CM. Depression and cardiovascular disease: mechanisms of interaction. *Biol Psychiatry*. 2003;54:248-261.

95. Glassman AH, O'Connor CM, Califf RM, et al. Sertraline treatment of major depression in patients with acute MI or unstable angina. *JAMA*. 2002;288:701-709.

96. Berkman LF, Blumenthal J, Burg M, et al. Effects of treating depression and low perceived social support on clinical events after myocardial infarction: the Enhancing Recovery in Coronary Heart Disease Patients (ENRICHD) Randomized Trial. *JAMA*. 2003;289:3106-3116.

97. Lesperance F, Frasure-Smith N, Koszycki D, et al. Effects of citalopram and interpersonal psychotherapy on depression in patients with coronary artery disease: the Canadian Cardiac Randomized Evaluation of Antidepressant and Psychotherapy Efficacy (CREATE) trial. *JAMA*. 2007;297:367-379.

98. Taylor CB, Youngblood ME, Catellier D, et al. Effects of antidepressant medication on morbidity and mortality in depressed patients after myocardial infarction. *Arch Gen Psychiatry*. 2005;62:792-798.

99. Serebruany VL, Gurbel PA, O'Connor CM. Platelet inhibition by sertraline and N-desmethylsertraline: a possible missing link between depression, coronary events, and mortality benefits of selective serotonin reuptake inhibitors. *Pharmacol Res*. 2001;43:453-462.

100. Katon W, Lin EH, Kroenke K. The association of depression and anxiety with medical symptom burden in patients with chronic medical illness. *Gen Hosp Psychiatry*. 2007;29:147-155.
101. Williams WR, Richards JP, Ameen JR, Davies J. Recurrent brief depression and personality traits in allergy, anxiety and premenstrual syndrome patients: A general practice survey. *Med Sci Monit*. 2007;13:CR118-124.
102. Lavoie KL, Bacon SL, Barone S, Cartier A, Ditto B, Labrecque M. What is worse for asthma control and quality of life: depressive disorders, anxiety disorders, or both? *Chest*. 2006;130:1039-1047.
103. Richardson LP, Lozano P, Russo J, McCauley E, Bush T, Katon W. Asthma symptom burden: relationship to asthma severity and anxiety and depression symptoms. *Pediatrics*. 2006;118:1042-1051.
104. Eisner MD, Katz PP, Lactao G, Iribarren C. Impact of depressive symptoms on adult asthma outcomes. *Ann Allergy Asthma Immunol*. 2005;94:566-574.
105. Baiardini I, Braido F, Giardini A, et al. Adherence to treatment: assessment of an unmet need in asthma. *J Investig Allergol Clin Immunol*. 2006;16:218-223.
106. Wainwright NW, Surtees PG, Wareham NJ, Harrison BD. Psychosocial factors and asthma in a community sample of older adults. *J Psychosom Res*. 2007;62:357-361.
107. Lavoie KL, Cartier A, Labrecque M, et al. Are psychiatric disorders associated with worse asthma control and quality of life in asthma patients? *Respir Med*. 2005;99:1249-1257.
108. Ekici A, Ekici M, Kara T, Keles H, Kocyigit P. Negative mood and quality of life in patients with asthma. *Qual Life Res*. 2006;15:49-56.
109. Covic T, Tyson G, Spencer D, Howe G. Depression in rheumatoid arthritis patients: demographic, clinical, and psychological predictors. *J Psychosom Res*. 2006;60:469-476.
110. Kothe R, Kohlmann T, Klink T, Ruther W, Klinger R. Impact of low back pain on functional limitations, depressed mood and quality of life in patients with rheumatoid arthritis. *Pain*. 2007;127:103-108.
111. Kozora E, Ellison MC, West S. Depression, fatigue, and pain in systemic lupus erythematosus (SLE): relationship to the American College of Rheumatology SLE neuropsychological battery. *Arthritis Rheum*. 2006;55:628-635.
112. Karassa FB, Magliano M, Isenberg DA. Suicide attempts in patients with systemic lupus erythematosus. *Ann Rheum Dis*. 2003;62:58-60.
113. Furst DE. Predictors of worsening clinical variables and outcomes in rheumatoid arthritis. *Rheum Dis Clin North Am*. 1994;20:309-319.
114. Chwastiak L, Ehde DM, Gibbons LE, Sullivan M, Bowen JD, Kraft GH. Depressive symptoms and severity of illness in multiple sclerosis: epidemiologic study of a large community sample. *Am J Psychiatry*. 2002;159:1862-1868.
115. Siegert RJ, Abernethy DA. Depression in multiple sclerosis: a review. *J Neurol Neurosurg Psychiatry*. 2005;76:469-475.
116. Feinstein A. An examination of suicidal intent in patients with multiple sclerosis. *Neurology*. 2002;59:674-678.
117. Stenager EN, Stenager E, Koch-Henriksen N, et al. Suicide and multiple sclerosis: an epidemiological investigation. *J Neurol Neurosurg Psychiatry*. 1992;55:542-545.
118. Sobel RM, Lotkowski S, Mandel S. Update on depression in neurologic illness: stroke, epilepsy, and multiple sclerosis. *Curr Psychiatry Rep*. 2005;7:396-403.
119. Gold SM, Irwin MR. Depression and immunity: inflammation and depressive symptoms in multiple sclerosis. *Neurol Clin*. 2006;24:507-519.
120. McGuigan C, Hutchinson M. Unrecognised symptoms of depression in a community-based population with multiple sclerosis. *J Neurol*. 2006;253:219-223.
121. Fountoulakis KN, Kantartzis S, Siamouli M, et al. Peripheral thyroid dysfunction in depression. *World J Biol Psychiatry*. 2006;7:131-137.
122. Carta MG, Loviselli A, Hardoy MC, et al. The link between thyroid autoimmunity (antithyroid peroxidase autoantibodies) with anxiety and mood disorders in the community: a field of interest for public health in the future. *BMC Psychiatry*. 2004;4:25.
123. Jones AL, Mowry BJ, Pender MP, Greer JM. Immune dysregulation and self-reactivity in schizophrenia: do some cases of schizophrenia have an autoimmune basis? *Immunol Cell Biol*. 2005;83:9-17.
124. Ronson A. Stress and allostatic load: perspectives in psycho-oncology. *Bull Cancer*. 2006;93:289-295.
125. Lloyd-Williams M. Difficulties in diagnosing and treating depression in the terminally ill cancer patient. *Postgrad Med J*. 2000;76:555-558.
126. Raison CL, Miller AH. Depression in cancer: new developments regarding diagnosis and treatment. *Biol Psychiatry*. 2003;54:283-294.
127. Pasquini M, Biondi M. Depression in cancer patients: a critical review. *Clin Pract Epidemol Ment Health*. 2007;3:2.
128. Bailey RK, Geyen DJ, Scott-Gurnell K, Hipolito MM, Bailey TA, Beal JM. Understanding and treating depression among cancer patients. *Int J Gynecol Cancer*. 2005;15:203-208.
129. Antoni MH, Lutgendorf SK, Cole SW, et al. The influence of bio-behavioural factors on tumour biology: pathways and mechanisms. *Nat Rev Cancer*. 2006;6:240-248.
130. Groenvold M, Petersen MA, Idler E, Bjorner JB, Fayers PM, Mouridsen HT. Psychological distress and fatigue predicted recurrence and survival in primary breast cancer patients. *Breast Cancer Res Treat*. 2007.
131. Wilson KG, Chochinov HM, Skirko MG, et al. Depression and anxiety disorders in palliative cancer care. *J Pain Symptom Manage*. 2007;33:118-129.
132. Holden RJ, Pakula IS, Mooney PA. An immunological model connecting the pathogenesis of stress, depression and carcinoma. *Med Hypotheses*. 1998;51:309-314.
133. Bone Health and Osteoporosis: A Report of the Surgeon General: US Department of Health and Human Services; Rockville, MD; 2004.
134. Michelson D, Stratakis C, Hill L, et al. Bone mineral density in women with depression. *N Engl J Med*. 1996;335:1176-1181.
135. Wong SY, Lau EM, Lynn H, et al. Depression and bone mineral density: is there a relationship in elderly Asian men? Results from Mr. Os (Hong Kong). *Osteoporos Int*. 2005;16:610-615.
136. Altindag O, Altindag A, Asoglu M, Gunes M, Soran N, Deveci Z. Relation of cortisol levels and bone mineral density among premenopausal women with major depression. *Int J Clin Pract*. 2007;61:416-420.
137. Mussolino ME. Depression and hip fracture risk: the NHANES I epidemiologic follow-up study. *Public Health Rep*. 2005;120:71-75.
138. Silverman SL, Shen W, Minshall ME, Xie S, Moses KH. Prevalence of depressive symptoms in postmenopausal women with low bone mineral density and/or prevalent vertebral fracture: results from the Multiple Outcomes of Raloxifene Evaluation (MORE) study. *J Rheumatol*. 2007;34:140-144.
139. Tolea MI, Black SA, Carter-Pokras OD, Kling MA. Depressive symptoms as a risk factor for osteoporosis and fractures in older Mexican American women. *Osteoporos Int*. 2007;18:315-322.
140. Gold DT, Solimeo S. Osteoporosis and depression: a historical perspective. *Curr Osteoporos Rep*. 2006;4:134-139.
141. Ilias I, Alesci S, Gold PW, Chrousos GP. Depression and osteoporosis in men: association or casual link? *Hormones (Athens)*. 2006;5:9-16.

142. Cizza G, Ravn P, Chrousos GP, Gold PW. Depression: a major, unrecognized risk factor for osteoporosis? *Trends Endocrinol Metab.* 2001;12:198-203.

143. Yazici KM, Akinci A, Sutcu A, Ozcakar L. Bone mineral density in premenopausal women with major depressive disorder. *Psychiatry Res.* 2003;117:271-275.

144. Kahl KG, Rudolf S, Stoeckelhuber BM, et al. Bone mineral density, markers of bone turnover, and cytokines in young women with borderline personality disorder with and without comorbid major depressive disorder. *Am J Psychiatry.* 2005;162:168-174.

145. Alesci S, Martinez PE, Kelkar S, et al. Major depression is associated with significant diurnal elevations in plasma interleukin-6 levels, a shift of its circadian rhythm, and loss of physiological complexity in its secretion: clinical implications. *J Clin Endocrinol Metab.* 2005;90:2522-2530.

146. Hossain P, Kawar B, El Nahas M. Obesity and diabetes in the developing world--a growing challenge. *N Engl J Med.* 2007;356:213-215.

147. Onyike CU, Crum RM, Lee HB, Lyketsos CG, Eaton WW. Is obesity associated with major depression? Results from the Third National Health and Nutrition Examination Survey. *Am J Epidemiol.* 2003;158:1139-1147.

148. Bornstein SR, Wong ML, Licinio J. 150 years of Sigmund Freud: What would Freud have said about the obesity epidemic? *Mol Psychiatry.* 2006;11:1070-1072.

149. Carpenter KM, Hasin DS, Allison DB, Faith MS. Relationships between obesity and DSM-IV major depressive disorder, suicide ideation, and suicide attempts: results from a general population study. *Am J Public Health.* 2000;90:251-257.

150. Lee ES, Kim YH, Beck SH, Lee S, Oh SW. Depressive mood and abdominal fat distribution in overweight premenopausal women. *Obes Res.* 2005;13:320-325.

151. Simon GE, Von Korff M, Saunders K, et al. Association between obesity and psychiatric disorders in the US adult population. *Arch Gen Psychiatry.* 2006;63:824-830.

152. Kress AM, Peterson MR, Hartzell MC. Association between obesity and depressive symptoms among U.S. Military active duty service personnel, 2002. *J Psychosom Res.* 2006;60:263-271.

153. Wadden TA, Butryn ML, Sarwer DB, et al. Comparison of psychosocial status in treatment-seeking women with class III vs. class I-II obesity. *Obesity (Silver Spring).* 2006;14 Suppl 2:90S-98S.

154. Kabir AA, Whelton PK, Khan MM, Gustat J, Chen W. Association of symptoms of depression and obesity with hypertension: the Bogalusa Heart Study. *Am J Hypertens.* 2006;19:639-645.

155. Moreira RO, Marca KF, Appolinario JC, Coutinho WF. Increased waist circumference is associated with an increased prevalence of mood disorders and depressive symptoms in obese women. *Eat Weight Disord.* 2007;12:35-40.

156. Ohayon MM. Epidemiology of depression and its treatment in the general population. *J Psychiatr Res.* 2007;41:207-213.

157. Tuthill A, Slawik H, O'Rahilly S, Finer N. Psychiatric co-morbidities in patients attending specialist obesity services in the UK. *Qjm.* 2006;99:317-325.

158. Vila G, Zipper E, Dabbas M, et al. Mental disorders in obese children and adolescents. *Psychosom Med.* 2004;66:387-394.

159. Bornstein SR, Schuppenies A, Wong ML, Licinio J. Approaching the shared biology of obesity and depression: the stress axis as the locus of gene-environment interactions. *Mol Psychiatry.* 2006;11:892-902.

160. Cani PD, Amar J, Iglesias MA, et al. Metabolic endotoxemia initiates obesity and insulin resistance. *Diabetes.* 2007;56:1761-1772.

161. Reichenberg A, Yirmiya R, Schuld A, et al. Cytokine-associated emotional and cognitive disturbances in humans. *Arch Gen Psychiatry.* 2001;58:445-452.

Section II

State of the Science in Assessment and Treatment

Antidepressant medications have provided a significant amount of relief over the past 50 years. The purpose of this monograph is not to deny the role and effectiveness of such drugs, but to address the large proportion (about 50%) of depressed patients who receive only partial or no benefit from them, for a variety of reasons. From the functional medicine perspective, many additional treatment options are available to address underlying dysfunctions that contribute to depression. Clinicians *can* substantially expand the universe of people who can be helped.

In this section, we will:

- Review the evidence underlying the urgent need for therapeutic approaches to depression in addition to (and in some cases in lieu of) pharmaceutical and psychotherapeutic ones.
- Examine aspects of the Functional Medicine Matrix Model for evidence of metabolic pathways and processes known to influence neuronal function and mood.
- Advance an inference based on these mechanisms and interconnections that remediating underlying dysfunctions will have a highly beneficial effect on many patients with depressive disorders, resulting in improved outcomes for a greater number of people.

In the final section (*Clinical Applications*), we will apply this complex array of possibilities to the challenge of effectively identifying and treating patients who need more help than is available from drug and psychotherapeutic treatments alone.

Chapter 4

Drug Treatments for Depression

Drug Classes and Mechanisms: A Brief Review

Since the first monoamine oxidase inhibitors (MAOIs) were developed in the 1950s, virtually all antidepressant drug advances have been based on enhancing monoamine neurotransmission.[1] Various mechanisms for accomplishing that goal have been explored, including blocking reuptake of serotonin/5-HT, dopamine, or norepinephrine; inhibiting metabolism of the neurotransmitters; blocking receptors that secondarily increase signal transduction through other receptors; increasing neuronal firing rate; and stimulating the release of neurotransmitters.[1] Although these strategies have shown clinical efficacy, they have failed to induce full recovery in more than 50% of patients, and the monamine hypothesis of affective disorders has failed to explain why it can take weeks for many patients to feel effects resulting from chemical changes that occur virtually immediately.[2]

Table 4.1 presents summary information about the most common classes of antidepressants in use today, drawn from a variety of sources. Table 4.2 provides dosages and more detailed information on side effects for specific medications.

Table 4.1*—Common Classes of Antidepressants

Class	Common Examples (name; brand name)	Primary Uses	Common Side Effects**	Cautions and Contraindications**
Norepinephrine reuptake inhibitor (NRI)	Desipramine (TCA/NRI); Norpramin® Reboxetine; Edronax®, Davedax®, or Vestra® Maprotiline; Ludiomil®	Depression Panic disorder	Tachycardia Insomnia Increased sweating Constipation Urinary hesitancy Dry mouth Blurry vision	ALL ANTIDEPRESSANTS now carry black box warnings regarding increased risk of suicide.
Selective serotonin/ 5-HT reuptake inhibitor (SSRI)	Fluoxetine; Prozac® Sertraline; Zoloft® Citalopram; Celexa® and escitalopram; Lexapro® Paroxetine; Paxil® (anticholinergic) Fluvoxamine; Luvox®	Depression Anxiety disorders Obsessive-compulsive disorder	Sexual dysfunction in up to 60% of patients Sedation or insomnia Nausea or diarrhea Anorexia Anxiety Nightmares, vivid dreams Headache Slight weight loss or gain	All may trigger manic episodes in bipolar disorder; some patients have reported suicidal thoughts/impulses. Should not be used with MAOIs (serotonin syndrome) and warfarin. May inhibit platelet function and prolong bleeding. Discontinuation syndrome.
Serotonin/5-HT-norepinephrine reuptake inhibitor (SNRI)	Imipramine; Tofranil® Amitriptyline; Elavil® Venlafaxine; Effexor® (dose-dependent inhibitor of dopamine reuptake) Duloxetine; Cymbalta® (weak inhibitor of dopamine reuptake)	Depression Panic disorder Duloxetine: diabetic peripheral neuropathy; generalized anxiety disorder	Nausea Hypertension or hypotension Dizziness Dry mouth or throat Fatigue Constipation Insomnia or somnolence Sexual dysfunction: loss of libido or anorgasmia	Must not be used with MAOIs; should be monitored carefully if used with TCAs, SSRIs, or major tranquilizers. Duloxetine may increase blood pressure; others may cause hypertension in high doses. Discontinuation syndrome.
Monamine oxidase inhibitor (MAOI)	Selegiline; Emsam® (patch) or Eldepryl® (greater safety in lower doses and greater tolerability than other MAOIs) Phenelzine; Nardil® Isocarboxazid; Marplan® Tranylcypromine; Parnate®	Depression Atypical depression Dysthymia	Dizziness Orthostatic hypotension Tachycardia Loss of libido Food reactions may generate dangerous rise in blood pressure, as well as headache, nausea, vomiting, psychotic symptoms, seizures, stroke, and coma	Severe reactions possible with tyramine-containing foods (e.g., aged cheeses, smoked and processed meats and fish, red wine, fava beans, ripe figs) and MSG-containing foods. Drug interactions highly likely with SSRIs (serotonin syndrome), OTC cold or allergy medicines, appetite suppressants, local anesthetics, insulin, amphetamines, cocaine, and drugs used to treat Parkinson's disease.

Drug Treatments for Depression

Class	Common Examples (name; brand name)	Primary Uses	Common Side Effects**	Cautions and Contraindications**
Tricyclic antidepressant (TCA)	Imipramine; Tofranil® Amitriptyline; Elavil® Amoxapine; Asendin® Nortriptyline; Aventyl® or Pamelor® Doxepin; Sinequan® Desipramine (TCA/NRI); Norpramin® Clomipramine; Anafranil® (for obsessive-compulsive disorder) Trimipramine; Surmontil® Protriptyline; Vivactil®	Depression Panic disorder Clomipramine: Obsessive-compulsive disorder	Drowsiness Tachycardia Anxiety Restlessness Dry mouth Constipation Urination problems Cognitive and memory problems Weight gain Increased sweating Dizziness Loss of libido Fatigue or weakness Blurred vision Nausea Muscle twitches	Can be dangerous, even fatal, if combined with other drugs. Can be lethal in high doses. Can aggravate narrow-angle glaucoma. Discontinuation syndrome can be attenuated via slow taper.
Receptor blocker (increased norepinephrine release and, indirectly, serotonin release)	Mirtazapine; Remeron®	Depression	Sleepiness or sedation Weight gain (with possible increases in cholesterol and triglycerides) Constipation Dizziness Orthostatic hypotension Fatigue Dry mouth Headache Increased appetite Disturbing dreams	Must not be used with MAOIs. Enhances effects of sedative drugs such as alcohol, tranquilizers, sleeping pills, barbiturates, buspirone, and other antidepressants. Overstimulating when mixed with venlafaxine
NRI + dopamine transmission inhibitor	Bupropion; Wellbutrin® (lowest risk for sexual side effects)	Depression	Insomnia Headache Tremors Nausea Irritability Agitation Hypertension Seizures in those at risk	Avoid prescribing for patients with any history of seizures, heavy alcohol use, eating disorders, head trauma, benzodiazepine withdrawal, or organic brain syndrome. Certain drugs can cause blood levels of bupropion to fall (barbiturates, phenytoin) or rise (cimetidine). May enhance effects of SSRIs and/or combat their sexual side effects. Must not be used with MAOIs.
Serotonin modulator	Trazodone; Desyrel® Nefazodone	Depression Insomnia	Dizziness Dry mouth Nausea Constipation Blurred vision Headache Fatigue Insomnia Confusion Anxiety	May enhance sedative effects of many other drugs and alcohol. Must not be used with MAOIs. Can increase blood levels of phenytoin and digoxin; may have unpredictable effects on warfarin. Nefazodone may cause liver dysfunction, up to actual failure. Trazodone may cause priapism in some men.

Table 4.2*—Dosages, Side Effects, Risks, and Special Uses of Antidepressants by Drug Name

Name	Daily Dose Range	Side Effects**	Special Uses/Risks**
Anafranil	25–75 mg 3x with food	A, B, c, S, w	D, OCD; possibly P, M, CP; Bld
Asendin	25–600 mg	A, b, c, S, w	D; uniquely effective for psychotic depression
Aventyl/Pamelor	25–150 mg	A, b, c, S, w	D; Bld; therapeutic window—level must be in specified range
Cymbalta	20–60 mg	T, n, h, i, a, S, w	D, Anx, SP, M, CP
Celexa	20–40 mg	b, n, h, i, S, w	D, Anx, SP, M, CP
Desyrel	25–600 mg	a, b, c, S, w	D, Anx, SP, M, CP
Effexor	25–125 mg 3x with food	N, T, a, b, h, i, S, w	D; mild benefit in ADD, P
Elavil	25–300 mg	A, B, C, S, w	D, U, M, CP; Bld
Emsam	6, 9, or 12 mg patch	H, I	D; dietary restrictions at moderate and higher doses
Lexapro	10–20 mg	b, n, h, i, S w	D, Anx, SP, M, CP
Ludiomil	25–225 mg	a, b, c, S, w	D; must raise dose slowly
Luvox	25–150 mg 2x	a, b, h ,n, S, w	OCD; probably P, CP, D
Nardil	15–105 mg	a, b, c, S, w	D, ADD, P, SP, Anx, CP
Nefazodone	100–300 mg 2x	N, a, b, c, S, w	D, Anx; fewer sexual side effects
Norpramin	25–350 mg	A, b, c, S, w	D, ADD; Bld
Parnate	10–90 mg	a, c, S, w	D (energizing); dietary restrictions
Paxil	5–800 mg	a, b, n, S, w	D; probably OCD, SP, SOM, CP, M
Pristiq (desvenlafaxine)	50 mg	c, n, i, S	D; delivers the metabolite of venlafaxine in its active form; not metabolized by the CYP 450 system, so may offer advantages for people on other medications
Prozac	5–80 mg	b, n, S, w	D, OCD, PMS
Sinequan	25–300 mg	A, B, C, S, w	D, Anx, U, CP, SOM; Bld
Surmontil	75–150 mg	A, B, C, S, w	D, Anx
Tofranil	25–300 mg	A, B, C, S, w	D, ADD, P, Anx; possibly OCD, SP, SOM; Bld
Vivactil	5–15 mg 3x	A, c, S, w	D (energizing); tolerated in patients with sleep apnea
Wellbutrin	75–450 mg in divided doses	A	D, ADD; no weight gain; risk of seizures in certain populations; must divide dosage or use extended release forms
Zoloft	25–200 mg	B, S, w	D; possibly useful in OCD, Anx, SP, CP

Key to Abbreviations in Table 4.2:

Upper case = significant effect, lower case = minor effect

- **A,a** = dry mouth, constipation, blurry vision
- **B,b** = sedation
- **C,c** = dizziness on standing
- **N,n** = nausea
- **H,h** = headache
- **I,i** = insomnia
- **T,t** = hypertension
- **D** = depression
- **ADD** = attention deficit disorder
- **Anx** = generalized anxiety disorder
- **CP** = chronic pain
- **M** = migraine
- **OCD** = obsessive-compulsive disorder
- **P** = panic disorder
- **S** = sexual side effects
- **SP** = social phobia
- **U** = ulcers
- **w** = weight gain
- **SOM** = somatization disorder
- **Bld** = monitoring of the level of medication in the patient's blood is necessary

Notes to Tables 4.1 and 4.2:

*While drugs here are separated into categories based on proposed mechanisms of action, structure, or drug names, the fact is that when any one neurotransmitter system is affected, others are secondarily affected to greater or lesser degrees, depending on dose, duration of use, and biochemical individuality. Effexor, for example, affects primarily serotonin at low doses, serotonin and norepinephrine at intermediate doses, and serotonin, norepinephrine, and dopamine at higher doses. Even highly selective serotonin medications (e.g., Paxil) will affect dopamine function secondarily, since all neurons are part of a larger neural network.

**Not all side effects, cautions, or contraindications reported in the literature are listed here, nor are those listed equally true of every drug in a particular class; clinicians should be completely informed about a particular drug before using it.

The antidepressant medications are useful in a broad range of disorders in addition to depression, including attention deficit disorder, panic disorder, generalized anxiety disorder, post-traumatic stress syndrome, somatization disorder, ulcers, migraine headache, and chronic pain syndromes. The fact that these medications are effective in such a seemingly diverse group of disorders is a likely indicator that there are common underlying abnormalities.

The antidepressant medications may be grouped according to:

- Chemical nature (i.e., by the number of rings in their molecular structure such as TCAs, heterocyclics; aminoketones)
- Mode of action (i.e., MAOIs, SSRIs, SNRIs)
- Side effects
- The chronology of their development (i.e., first, second, third generation)

The grouping by side effects parallels the grouping by chronology and is most practical for the nonpsychiatric mental health provider. The development of the antidepressant medications occurred in 3 waves, or generations. In general, each succeeding generation has had fewer side effects and has been more selective in chemical action but has not improved in efficacy. Overall, no antidepressant seems to be more effective than others for the treatment of depression when tested in large-scale studies. In individual cases, it is common for a patient to respond to one agent and not another. This may be related to the probability that there are subtypes of depression, each affecting different neurotransmitters to different degrees.

The First Generation of Antidepressants

Developed in the late 1950s, these first-generation antidepressants included the tricyclics (so called because they have 3 rings in their structure) and the MAOIs. The tricyclic antidepressants (TCAs) have many side effects due to their wide-ranging biological actions, and they are almost impossible for some people to tolerate. This problem helped to spur the development of the second- and third-generation antidepressants. However, first-generation medications are still very useful, despite the newer, better-tolerated medications now on the market.

The TCA group includes 2 parent compounds: Elavil (amitriptyline, the first antidepressant) and Tofranil (imipramine). The remaining members of this group are either breakdown products of a parent compound or have subtle changes in their chemical structure that confer different clinical properties. These other TCAs include Asendin (amoxapine), Aventyl/Pamelor (nortriptyline, a breakdown product of Elavil), Norpramin (desipramine, the breakdown product of imipramine), Anafranil (clomipramine), Sinequan (doxepin), Surmontil (trimipramine), and Vivactil (protriptyline).

Historically, the most commonly used MAOIs included Nardil (phenelzine) and Parnate (tranylcypromine), although with the introduction of the selegiline patch (Emsam) this is rapidly changing. These medications are quite effective in the treatment of depression, panic disorder, and various types of anxiety but—except in the case of Emsam at low doses—they require strict adherence to a special diet (no foods with tyramine or MSG) in order to prevent the risk of sudden elevation of blood pressure (a hypertensive episode); in rare cases, this can lead to stroke or death, an event that was more common in the 1960s before awareness of the need for dietary precautions. MAOIs should be used only in responsible, compliant individuals who can closely follow such a diet and comply with instructions about how to deal with a hypertensive crisis. In nearly every study comparing the efficacy of Nardil against other antidepressants, Nardil is equal to the other agents as an antidepressant and superior as an antianxiety agent.[3] It is also very useful in panic disorder and social phobia,[4, 5] as well as atypical depression.

Currently, new agents are being researched that can work as MAOIs without the need for dietary restrictions. These agents work on a reversible inhibition of the same enzyme, rather than the current irreversible inhibition of the enzyme, which can be undone only slowly as the body manufactures new quantities of the enzyme. They are called reversible inhibitors of MAO A (RIMAs) and include 2 drugs in the experimental phase: brofaromine and moclobemide. Moclobemide is available overseas but is not approved in the United States.

The Second Generation of Antidepressants

This group, first marketed in the early 1980s, includes chemically unrelated medications that generally have fewer side effects than the TCAs. Included in this group are Asendin (amoxapine), Ludiomil (maprotiline), and Desyrel (trazodone). Asendin, a second-generation TCA of the dibenzoxazepine class, seems to be particularly useful in psychotic depression,[4] as one of its breakdown products has antipsychotic effects. Ludiomil is very potent as a norepinephrine agent.[5] Desyrel, often used as a sleep aid,[6] can cause sustained and painful erection in males (priapism) and therefore should be avoided in men; it is, however, useful in patients with epilepsy, as it does not lower the seizure threshold.

The Third Generation of Antidepressants

SSRIs and SNRIs are distinguished by fewer side effects and a relative selectivity of action. In the late 1980s, these compounds brought about a revolution in psychopharmacology, which ultimately allowed managed care companies to shift the treatment of most depressive disorders to primary care physicians and to limit the use of psychotherapy. It also became possible to treat the more subtle forms of depression, such as chronically anxious, low-grade depressions (atypical depression), without the severe side effects of the earlier medications. Prior to the advent of these medications, the major decisions and life courses of these patients were altered on a subtle scale by their hyperresponsiveness to and fears of separation, avoidance of novelty and risk, chronic procrastination, and lack of initiative and assertiveness. In these patients, treatment used to involve the MAOIs, which are generally more dangerous due to the risk of acute hypertensive crisis provoked by tyramine- or MSG-containing foods.

Included in the third generation of SSRIs are Prozac (fluoxetine), Zoloft (sertraline), Paxil (paroxetine), Luvox (fluvoxamine), Celexa (citalopram), and Lexapro (escitalopram). Wellbutrin (bupropion), Cymbalta (duloxetine), and Effexor (venlafaxine) are also third-generation medications with reduced side effects, but they are different from the SSRIs in that they have mild serotonin actions as well as norepinephrine actions (Cymbalta and Effexor) or strictly dopaminergic and noradrenergic actions (Wellbutrin).

The increased tolerability of these third-generation medications has expanded the scope of psychopharmacology, bringing into focus the nature of personality and its chemical, genetic, and environmental origins. Researchers are examining this interaction between inborn biological response styles and environmental influences. Yet some challenging questions have been raised: Is it morally, socially, and ethically correct to alter the biological response style of a person? What are the personal and social consequences of such interventions when applied to a large and growing segment of the population? Have we arrived at the brave new world where false happiness can be attained with a pill? Does suffering serve a purpose? What about creativity and art? Where would society be without individuals such as Mozart and Van Gogh? What if they had taken Prozac? What factors in a culture lead to a rising demand for such chemical interventions?

The recent controversy in the media regarding the safety of these medications (that is, whether they cause suicidal or homicidal behavior) is in large measure an artifact of a healthcare system that has compressed psychiatric evaluation into the very briefest of times (e.g., 20-45 minutes). The fact is that any antidepressant, any psychiatric medication, and many nonpsychiatric medications may cause psychotic (suicidal or homicidal) behavior. Any minor tranquilizer can cause depression or agitation. *These medications require careful evaluation of the patient and close follow-up in the context of good patient-physician communication.*

Antidepressant Outcomes and Limitations of the Evidence

There are many limitations to the use of drugs. Side effects (see Tables 4.1 and 4.2), drug interactions, latency (length of time for treatment to become effective), cost, variable or unpredictable individual responses, insurance-approved drug lists that fail to consider differential prescribing, and the high frequency of partially responsive and treatment-resistant depression are all issues that should make us persist in our search for other answers. Lack of compliance due to side effects is such a major issue that it alone could be a sufficient impetus for pursuing nondrug approaches: up to 70% of patients taking antidepressants are noncompliant, and side effects are the most common reason.[7]

Despite the variety of drugs available for the treatment of depression, there are several difficulties in ascertaining the true efficacy of such drugs across all patients, even when we look at the most credible evidence:

- **Inadequate criteria for efficacy** — Until very recently, even the most rigorous drug trials used response rather than recovery (or full remission) as the standard for success.[8] The definition most widely used for reporting a positive outcome in drug trials is a 50% or greater reduction in symptoms, based on a validated rating scale of depression severity, such as the Hamilton Depression Rating Scale (HAM-D).[9] A patient whose symptoms have diminished by 50% or 60% is not, however, a depression-free individual. If a person has a HAM-D score of 36 (normal = <10), indicating severe depression, and is treated with medication that lowers her score to 18, she still has a severe depression, despite the fact that the score has been cut in half. In addition, a large proportion of the overall response to an antidepressant may be the result of a placebo response, which is added to the pharmacological response.[10]

- **Variety in rating scales** — The considerable variety of scales used to evaluate treatment outcomes makes an apples-to-apples comparison of outcomes difficult. The scales often don't measure the same elements in the same ways, and some were developed for other purposes (such as screening) and were not originally intended as outcome measures at all. For example, the 2 scales most widely used in antidepressant efficacy trials (the HAM-D and the Montgomery-Asberg Depression Rating Scale, or MADRS) have some important differences:
  - The HAM-D assesses primarily the severity of depressive symptoms; the MADRS was designed primarily to detect mood changes in patients treated with antidepressants.[11]
  - The HAM-D has a heavy emphasis on sleep-related symptoms, while the MADRS does not.[12] Using the HAM-D can bias the outcome in favor of drugs that have a sedative effect.[13]
  - The use of different cutoff scores "considerably influences the percentage of patients determined to be in remission."[14]

- **Limited effectiveness** — Response rates—*not recovery or full remission rates*—in randomized controlled trials (RCTs) at 6 to 8 weeks are in the 50–65% range among all antidepressant drugs, and remission rates in pooled data range from 45% (Effexor) to 35% (SSRIs).[9] We must ask, therefore, where that leaves the remaining 55–65% of patients?
  - From 1000 patients, assume you have 500 responders and 500 nonresponders.
  - Among the 500 responders, some lower number (350 to 450) will actually be in remission, and the rest will have at least a 50% reduction in symptoms.
  - Out of 1000 people, then, you have 500 who are not helped, 100 who are partially helped, and around 400 who are in remission.
  - The obvious conclusion from even a casual analysis is that 50% to 60% of depressed people from the RCT patient pool still desperately need access to treatments other than (or in addition to) antidepressant drugs.

- **Difficulty extrapolating from RCT patients to community-based care** — More than 50% of research-qualified patients do not get well within 2 months.[9] Clearly, many patients in research trials are helped—perhaps 35% to 45% are in remission. However, we don't know whether that figure holds true in clinical practice. Screening for participation in drug trials creates a patient pool that rarely resembles the patient population seen in normal clinical care, thus making generalizations problematic. The type of depression (atypical, melancholic, dysthymic, etc.) is usually not defined for drug trials, and patients with many common comorbidities are routinely excluded from the pool. In addition, diagnostic criteria for participants in drug trials have varied substantially over the years, further complicating the effort to distinguish which drugs work with which conditions.[13] In a major 2006 review of antidepressant therapy, Zetin et al[9] provided an excellent discussion of the difficulty in mapping RCT outcomes to real patients. Unfortunately, their solution is to call for more RCTs on drugs. We strongly advocate looking beyond pharmaceuticals for additional solutions, a recommendation that is based on the large body of research presented in this monograph.

Strategies for Enhancing Antidepressant Effectiveness

The search for strategies to enhance the effectiveness of antidepressant drugs has taken many different turns; we will review here only the most widely used. It's important to note that all of these are, essentially, *off-label uses* since the FDA has not recognized any enhancement strategies for antidepressants.

Augmentation

This strategy involves adding another medication to the antidepressant drug. Among the most commonly prescribed augmentation medications are:

Lithium — A substantial number of controlled trials have reported that lithium is effective as an augmentation strategy.[15] Most of these studies were done with TCAs augmented by lithium; a meta-analysis in 1999 reported that "with respect to efficacy, lithium augmentation is the first-choice treatment procedure for depressed patients who fail to respond to antidepressant monotherapy."[16] However, at least 2 studies published subsequent to the meta-analysis studied the augmentation effect using SSRIs or SNRIs with lithium and did not replicate the TCA results.[17, 18] It has been hypothesized that perhaps bipolar patients were included in studies done in the 1980s, thereby confounding the results for patients with unipolar depression.[19] A study of non-refractory patients, involving more subjects than the total pool in the meta-analysis (142 vs. 110), found the potentiation effect of lithium to be less convincing (not statistically significant at day 11) and to disappear by the end of 6 weeks of treatment.[20] *Lithium has been shown to be the most efficacious medication in terms of suicide prevention.*[21]

Thyroid (high-dose T3/Cytomel®/T4) — All controlled studies of thyroid hormone augmentation with treatment-resistant patients have been done with TCAs; positive effects have been reported in some, although not all, studies, and at least 6 studies reported an accelerated clinical response (although in patients with non-refractory depression).[19] Studies of treatment-resistant patients treated with SSRIs plus T3 or T4 showed promising results,[22-25] but no controlled studies have as yet been done. Overall, there is good evidence to support the effectiveness of T3 (and also T4[26-28]) as augmentation therapy for some patients who do not achieve a good response to initial drug treatment. However, most of these results are for improved response, not full remission. Generally, clinicians prefer to use T3 in high doses (25–50 µg/d) at initiation of treatment, although there is no clear consensus.

Folic acid — There is growing evidence of a relationship between low folate levels, depression, and response to antidepressant drugs.[29] A 2003 Cochrane collaboration report concluded that "the limited available evidence suggests folate may have a potential role as a supplement to other treatment for depression."[30] Not only do many studies document low folate levels in depressed patients,[31] but low folate is also associated with a poor response to antidepressant treatment[32, 33] and greater duration of the depressive episode.[29] One study used folate alone to treat depression, and another showed superior response rates and fewer side effects when folate was added.[34] Although much more research is needed to clarify the underlying mechanisms that connect folate levels to depression and treatment response, there have been serious recommendations to treat all depressed patients with folate during both acute and maintenance treatment.[31, 33] Recommendations of 800 µg to 2 mg have been made.[31-33]

Novel antipsychotics — In a brief discussion of 3 studies that combined a novel antipsychotic (e.g., risperidone or olanzapine) with an SSRI, Shelton reported some positive outcomes in treatment-resistant patients.[15]

Combination Therapy

This strategy involves adding a second antidepressant drug to the treatment program. The antidepressants are usually from different classes and are both given at full doses. The combination strategy is commonly used when drug monotherapy produces an inadequate response, but it has also been used to speed up the onset of the antidepressant effect. It is not known whether the efficacy of combining antidepressants is due to some sort of synergy between the 2 medications or simply from exposure to another antidepressant.[19] Common combinations include SSRIs with Wellbutrin, BuSpar® (buspirone), Remeron, mianserin, Edronax/Davedax/Vestra, Strattera® (atomoxetine), nefazodone/trazodone, TCAs, or dopamine receptor agonists. For a review of studies on this strategy, see Fava and Rush.[19]

Switching Strategy

Switching strategy involves selecting a different antidepressant within the same or a different class of drugs after an inadequate response to the first drug, usually an SSRI. Because the "large majority of depressed patients fail to remit on the first antidepressant prescribed,"[35] switching strategies are of considerable importance. Unfortunately, there is little evidence on which clinicians can base their decisions when deciding on a second drug when the first fails to relieve a patient's depression. In 2006, Ruhé et al published a systematic review[36] of the literature regarding the switching options; articles were found on the following switching options: a second SSRI, TCAs, mianserin, Remeron, nefazodone, Effexor, Wellbutrin, Edronax/Davedax/Vestra, and MAOIs. Switching to any of these antidepressants was found to have an approximately 50% chance of response, but a direct comparison of rates across the predominantly open studies was methodologically not justified.

In 2007, reports from the STAR-D (Sequenced Treatment Alternatives to Relieve Depression) study began to appear. This large prospective study involving a series of RCTs found "no differences in remission rates or times to remission among medication switch or among medication augmentation strategies at any treatment level."[37]

References

1. Delgado PL. How antidepressants help depression: Mechanisms of action and clinical response. *J Clin Psychiatry*. 2004;65:25-30.
2. Strohle A, Holsboer F. Stress responsive neurohormones in depression and anxiety. *Pharmacopsychiatry*. 2003;36 Suppl 3:S207-214.
3. Birkenhager TK, van den Broek WW, Mulder PG, Bruijn JA, Moleman P. Efficacy and tolerability of tranylcypromine versus phenelzine: a double-blind study in antidepressant-refractory depressed inpatients. *J Clin Psychiatry*. 2004;65:1505-1510.
4. Rothschild AJ. Challenges in the treatment of depression with psychotic features. *Biol Psychiatry*. 2003;53:680-690.
5. Humble M. Noradrenaline and serotonin reuptake inhibition as clinical principles: a review of antidepressant efficacy. *Acta Psychiatr Scand Suppl*. 2000;402:28-36.
6. Lieberman JA. Update on the safety considerations in the management of insomnia with hypnotics: incorporating modified-release formulations into primary care. *Prim Care Companion J Clin Psychiatry*. 2007;9:25-31.
7. Khawam EA, Laurencic G, Malone DA, Jr. Side effects of antidepressants: an overview. *Cleve Clin J Med*. 2006;73:351-353, 356-361.
8. Lam RW, Kennedy SH. Evidence-based strategies for achieving and sustaining full remission in depression: focus on metaanalyses. *Can J Psychiatry*. 2004;49:17S-26S.
9. Zetin M, Hoepner CT, Bjornson L. Rational antidepressant selection: Applying evidence-based medicine to complex real-world patients. *Psychopharmacol Bull*. 2006;39:38-104.
10. Alexopoulos GS, Kanellopoulos D, Murphy C, Gunning-Dixon F, Katz R, Heo M. Placebo response and antidepressant response. *Am J Geriatr Psychiatry*. 2007;15:149-158.
11. Zimmerman M, Posternak MA, Chelminski I. Defining remission on the Montgomery-Asberg depression rating scale. *J Clin Psychiatry*. 2004;65:163-168.
12. Gelenberg AJ, Chesen CL. How fast are antidepressants? *J Clin Psychiatry*. 2000;61:712-721.
13. Montgomery SA. Why do we need new and better antidepressants? *Int Clin Psychopharmacol*. 2006;21 Suppl 1:S1-S10.
14. Zimmerman M, Posternak MA, Chelminski I. Implications of using different cut-offs on symptom severity scales to define remission from depression. *Int Clin Psychopharmacol*. 2004;19:215-220.
15. Shelton RC. The use of antidepressants in novel combination therapies. *J Clin Psychiatry*. 2003;64 Suppl 2:14-18.
16. Bauer M, Dopfmer S. Lithium augmentation in treatment-resistant depression: meta-analysis of placebo-controlled studies. *J Clin Psychopharmacol*. 1999;19:427-434.
17. Fava M, Alpert J, Nierenberg A, et al. Double-blind study of high-dose fluoxetine versus lithium or desipramine augmentation of fluoxetine in partial responders and nonresponders to fluoxetine. *J Clin Psychopharmacol*. 2002;22:379-387.
18. Nierenberg AA, Papakostas GI, Petersen T, et al. Lithium augmentation of nortriptyline for subjects resistant to multiple antidepressants. *J Clin Psychopharmacol*. 2003;23:92-95.

19. Fava M, Rush AJ. Current status of augmentation and combination treatments for major depressive disorder: a literature review and a proposal for a novel approach to improve practice. *Psychother Psychosom.* 2006;75:139-153.

20. Januel D, Poirier MF, D'Alche-Biree F, Dib M, Olie JP. Multicenter double-blind randomized parallel-group clinical trial of efficacy of the combination clomipramine (150 mg/day) plus lithium carbonate (750 mg/day) versus clomipramine (150 mg/day) plus placebo in the treatment of unipolar major depression. *J Affect Disord.* 2003;76:191-200.

21. Guzzetta F, Tondo L, Centorrino F, Baldessarini RJ. Lithium treatment reduces suicide risk in recurrent major depressive disorder. *J Clin Psychiatry.* 2007;68:380-383.

22. Aronson R, Offman HJ, Joffe RT, Naylor CD. Triiodothyronine augmentation in the treatment of refractory depression. A meta-analysis. *Arch Gen Psychiatry.* 1996;53:842-848.

23. Iosifescu DV, Nierenberg AA, Mischoulon D, et al. An open study of triiodothyronine augmentation of selective serotonin reuptake inhibitors in treatment-resistant major depressive disorder. *J Clin Psychiatry.* 2005;66:1038-1042.

24. Abraham G, Milev R, Stuart Lawson J. T3 augmentation of SSRI resistant depression. *J Affect Disord.* 2006;91:211-215.

25. Lifschytz T, Segman R, Shalom G, et al. Basic mechanisms of augmentation of antidepressant effects with thyroid hormone. *Curr Drug Targets.* 2006;7:203-210.

26. Baumgartner A. Thyroxine and the treatment of affective disorders: an overview of the results of basic and clinical research. *Int J Neuropsychopharmacol.* 2000;3:149-165.

27. Lojko D, Rybakowski JK. l-thyroxine augmentation of serotonergic antidepressants in female patients with refractory depression. *J Affect Disord.* 2007.

28. Joffe RT. Is the thyroid still important in major depression? *J Psychiatry Neurosci.* 2006;31:367-368.

29. Alpert JE, Mischoulon D, Nierenberg AA, Fava M. Nutrition and depression: focus on folate. *Nutrition.* 2000;16:544-546.

30. Taylor MJ, Carney S, Geddes J, Goodwin G. Folate for depressive disorders. *Cochrane Database Syst Rev.* 2003:CD003390.

31. Young SN. Folate and depression--a neglected problem. *J Psychiatry Neurosci.* 2007;32:80-82.

32. Coppen A, Bolander-Gouaille C. Treatment of depression: time to consider folic acid and vitamin B12. *J Psychopharmacol.* 2005;19:59-65.

33. Abou-Saleh MT, Coppen A. Folic acid and the treatment of depression. *J Psychosom Res.* 2006;61:285-287.

34. Taylor MJ, Carney SM, Goodwin GM, Geddes JR. Folate for depressive disorders: systematic review and meta-analysis of randomized controlled trials. *J Psychopharmacol.* 2004;18:251-256.

35. Carvalho AF, Cavalcante JL, Castelo MS, Lima MC. Augmentation strategies for treatment-resistant depression: a literature review. *J Clin Pharm Ther.* 2007;32:415-428.

36. Ruhe HG, Huyser J, Swinkels JA, Schene AH. Switching antidepressants after a first selective serotonin reuptake inhibitor in major depressive disorder: a systematic review. *J Clin Psychiatry.* 2006;67:1836-1855.

37. Warden D, Rush AJ, Trivedi MH, Fava M, Wisniewski SR. The STAR*D Project results: a comprehensive review of findings. *Curr Psychiatry Rep.* 2007;9:449-459.

Chapter 5

Psychotherapy and Other Conventional Treatments

Psychotherapy

Cognitive-Behavioral Therapy

The premise of cognitive-behavioral therapy (CBT), which was developed more than 40 years ago, is that depressive symptoms stem from dysfunctional beliefs and thought processes as a result of early learning experiences. These beliefs may lie dormant until they are activated by a situation or event that has specific meaning for the individual. For many patients, identifying and challenging negative automatic thoughts is the main focus of CBT.[1]

Several studies have shown the effectiveness of CBT in reducing symptoms and relapse rates, with or without medication, for a variety of psychiatric disorders including depression.[2] In a recent review[3] of CBT outcome meta-analyses from 1967 to 2003, large effect sizes (grand mean = 0.90) were found for CBT in unipolar depression, generalized anxiety disorder, panic disorder with or without agoraphobia, social phobia, and childhood depressive and anxiety disorders. CBT was as effective as medication for moderate to severe depression in a 2005 placebo-controlled trial; in addition, relapse rates were 40% for CBT vs. 46% for medication after 16 weeks.[4] In a study of continuation treatment for residual depressive symptoms, the combination of CBT and fluoxetine failed to yield any significant benefit in symptoms or relapse rates over fluoxetine alone.[5] However, other studies have reported that CBT lessens the chance of relapse and recurrence up to a year after therapy ends.[6-8] Fava et al[9] showed that sequential use of CBT after successful pharmacotherapy improved long-term outcome in recurrent depression; after antidepressants were discontinued, those assigned to CBT for residual symptoms had a 40% relapse rate vs. 90% for those assigned to clinical management alone.

Interpersonal Therapy

Though not as established or as studied as CBT, interpersonal therapy (IPT) has shown similar treatment outcomes. This form of psychotherapy is based on the premise that depression occurs in a social and interpersonal context; it focuses on present rather than past relationships and on interpersonal rather than intrapsychic processes.[1]

IPT alone has been shown to be more effective than either medication alone[10] or a combination of IPT and medication,[11] although some evidence has been contradictory.[12] A separate study suggests that IPT may decrease the potency of life events in provoking recurrence of depression in women.[13] A 2007 investigation of maintenance treatment for women with recurrent depression found that IPT monotherapy prevented relapse in patients who achieved remission with IPT alone, but that it was less effective in those who required the addition of pharmacotherapy in initial treatment.[14]

Other Types of Psychotherapy

Recent studies also have provided support for the efficacy of problem-solving treatment and group psycho-education.[15, 16]

Psychotherapy in Combination with Medication

Overall, investigations of whether psychotherapy combined with antidepressant therapy is associated with a higher improvement rate than drug treatment alone have shown mixed results. At least 2 literature reviews[17, 18] support the superiority of combination therapy and indicate that the addition of psychotherapy improves adherence to treatment.[17] However, other studies have shown that the advantage of combination therapy varied with severity and chronicity of depression. For example, in a 2007 meta-analysis of 7 studies, "Combined therapy outperformed psychotherapy in moderate chronic depression only. No differences were found in mild and moderate non-chronic depression. No data were found for mild chronic depression and for severe depression."[19]

Studies also have reported the following:

- Combination therapy is the most effective option in chronic major depression, but the evidence is mixed in dysthmia, reported a 2003 review.[20]
- Among patients with major depression, combination therapy was much more effective than medication alone or CBT alone; however, among those with depression and a history of early childhood trauma, CBT alone was superior to medication alone, and the combination was only marginally superior to CBT alone.[21]
- Combination therapy was more effective than medication alone for depressed patients with personality disorders, but this was untrue in depressed patients without personality disorders.[22]
- In geriatric patients with recurrent major depression, combination treatment with IPT and nortriptyline was the optimal strategy for preventing relapse.[23]

Other Treatments for Depression

Electroconvulsive Therapy

Strong evidence shows that electroconvulsive therapy (ECT) is effective in major depressive episodes, especially those involving psychotic depression, and that it also prevents relapse and reduces the acute risk of suicide.[24-26] In 2003, *The Lancet* published a systematic review and meta-analysis[27] with the following conclusions:

- Real ECT is significantly more effective than simulated ECT.
- Treatment with ECT is significantly more effective than pharmacotherapy.
- Bilateral ECT is more effective than unipolar ECT.
- Cognitive impairment after ECT consists mostly of temporary anterograde and retrograde amnesia.

A separate review[25] reported that bilateral ECT produces greater impairment than unilateral ECT and that higher-energy treatment produces greater impairment than lower energy. Yet American Psychiatric Association practice guidelines note the "diminished efficacy of barely suprathreshold electrical stimulation with right unilateral electrode placement and a corresponding need to administer right unilateral ECT at stimulus intensities that are at least 6 times the initial seizure threshold."[28]

In a study conducted by the Consortium for Research in ECT (CORE), thrice-weekly bilateral ECT produced remission rates of 75% in 253 patients with major depressive disorder,[29] and in a second CORE study, relapse rates were similar for both continuation ECT (37.1%) and a combination of lithium and nortriptyline (31.6%).[30] In an earlier study published in *JAMA*, 55% of 290 patients with major depression achieved remission after thrice-weekly ECT treatments; all patients were given right unilateral ECT and those who did not show substantial improvement within 5 to 8 treatments were switched to bilateral ECT. Eighty-four of the remitting patients were randomized to 3 continuation groups (none including ECT), and relapse rates were 84% for placebo, 60% for nortriptyline, and 39% for a combination of nortriptyline and lithium.[31]

After more than 70 years of clinical experience, the therapeutic mechanism of ECT has still not been established. One hypothesis is derived from data showing vegetative dysfunction and abnormal hormone regulation in mood disorders. "These functions are normalized with repeated seizure inductions, perhaps through the release of extraordinary amounts of brain peptides and subsequent systemic hormonal changes."[24] A 2007 study found that plasma levels of brain-derived neurotrophic factor (BDNF) increased significantly in individuals receiving ECT for major depression, suggesting that BDNF may serve as a marker of the effects of this therapy.[32]

Vagal Nerve Stimulation

In 2005, the FDA approved vagal nerve stimulation (VNS) as a treatment for refractory depression. This technique, also used for epilepsy in the United States and Europe, uses a small generator implanted in the chest to deliver electrical impulses to the left vagus nerve in the neck at regular intervals. Clinicians are able to adjust stimulation parameters noninvasively using a telemetric wand linked to a handheld personal digital assistant. This therapy was first investigated for depression after the discovery of mood improvements in epilepsy patients after VNS treatments. PET imaging demonstrated reductions in the metabolic activity of the amygdala, hippocampus, and cingulate gyrus.[33]

So far, research indicates that the efficacy of VNS increases over time and that it is most useful for chronic, long-term therapy. For example, in a short-term trial of treatment-resistant unipolar depression and depressed-phase bipolar disorder patients, all of whom continued on a stable medication regimen, response rates were 15.2% for VNS and 10.0% for sham treatment after 12 weeks.[34] However, both groups were then given active treatment, and rates of response and remission doubled between 3 and 12 months.[35] Remission rates were found to be significantly higher with VNS therapy plus treatment as usual (13.2%) than in a control group who received only treatment as usual (3.2%).[36] See Nemeroff et al[33] for a discussion of VNS mechanisms of effect and additional research results.

Transcranial Magnetic Stimulation

Transcranial magnetic stimulation (TMS) is a 20-year-old technique used to evaluate excitatory/inhibitory intracortical circuits, the physiology and pathophysiology of various neuropsychiatric diseases, and the mechanisms of brain plasticity and of neuroactive drugs.[37] Repetitive TMS (rTMS) induces electrical currents in focal areas of the cerebral cortex, and it is hypothesized that these currents can transiently activate or inhibit focal cortical areas and thus influence behavior.[38] This technique has received attention as a possible treatment method for supplementing or even replacing drug treatment and ECT in depression. However, after initial enthusiasm, effect sizes have been smaller in more recent trials.[39-41] While some researchers feel that inadequate binding to placebo has harmed results,[1] meta-analyses nevertheless indicate that rTMS is still an experimental modality. It is not clear whether rTMS is significantly better than sham rTMS.[42, 43] Although scores on depression rating scales decreased after short courses of rTMS, significant remission is rare.[44]

A potential side effect of TMS is the induction of seizures. While it has been difficult until recently to reliably induce seizures with this method, there have been some successful trials of magnetic seizure therapy (MST) as a treatment in depression.[45-47] Notably, MST is associated with fewer side effects and more rapid recovery of cognitive function than ECT, although it has not been shown to be a superior treatment.

Deep Brain Stimulation

This treatment, used in Parkinson's disease, essential tremor, and dystonia, involves the surgical implantation of a "brain pacemaker" to send electrical impulses to certain parts of the brain. Evidence of usefulness in depression is scarce, but striking responses have been shown in at least 2 small studies.[48, 49] Successful trials of deep brain stimulation have also been conducted in refractory obsessive-compulsive and anxiety disorders.[1]

New Directions

Drug treatments with novel mechanisms of action are being studied. These future antidepressants may include:

- Hormone-linked treatments such as estrogen replacement therapy (the estradiol patch was effective in treating postmenopausal/perimenopausal depression,[50-52] relieving symptoms of depression in healthy older women,[92] and relieving depression in women following mini-gastric bypass[53]) and the steroid antagonist mifepristone (RU-486 or C-1073)
- Novel antagonist peptides such as corticotropin-releasing factor (CRF), neurokinins, and injectable penta-peptides
- Agents that affect glutamate neurotransmission,[54] such as lamotrigine (used for bipolar depression), which inhibits voltage-dependent sodium channels, resulting in decreased release of the excitatory neurotransmitters glutamate and aspartate

Future possibilities for nonpharmacological depression treatment include mindfulness-based cognitive therapy, acupuncture, and bright light therapy. Although research on these interventions and their specific effects is still in its infancy, all three have shown some success.

- Mindfulness describes a meditative approach that entails nonjudgmental, detached awareness of thoughts and feelings. As described by Kabat-Zinn,[55] this type of meditation can abate or short-circuit the fight-or-flight response and increase the capacity to bear physical pain and emotional stress. Current evidence from 2 randomized trials suggests that, for patients with 3 or more previous depressive episodes, mindfulness-based cognitive therapy has an additive benefit to usual care.[56]
- Electro-acupuncture combined with paroxetine had better clinical efficacy than paroxetine alone, with milder adverse reaction and quicker initiation of effect, in a recent trial.[57] In another study, laser acupuncture produced a greater reduction in depressive symptoms than simulated acupuncture.[58] Still another study showed rates of response and relapse with acupuncture that were comparable to those of conventional treatments.[59] However, the data do not support acupuncture as a monotherapy.[60]
- Light therapy provides exposure to specific wavelengths of light using lasers, LEDs, fluorescent lamps, dichroic lamps, or very bright, full-spectrum light. The efficacy of this therapy for winter depression has been established for some time, but recently it has been recognized as a valuable adjuvant to medication in patients with nonseasonal depression.[61, 62] A 2004 Cochrane review[63] noted that light therapy is most effective when administered in the first week of treatment, in the morning, and in sleep deprivation responders.

Other new avenues for treatment currently being explored are yoga,[64] osteopathic manipulative treatment,[65] and massage, with or without aromatherapy.[66]

References

1. Ebmeier KP, Donaghey C, Steele JD. Recent developments and current controversies in depression. *Lancet.* 2006;367:153-167.
2. Beck AT. The current state of cognitive therapy: a 40-year retrospective. *Arch Gen Psychiatry.* 2005;62:953-959.
3. Butler AC, Chapman JE, Forman EM, Beck AT. The empirical status of cognitive-behavioral therapy: a review of meta-analyses. *Clin Psychol Rev.* 2006;26:17-31.

4.   DeRubeis RJ, Hollon SD, Amsterdam JD, et al. Cognitive therapy vs medications in the treatment of moderate to severe depression. *Arch Gen Psychiatry.* 2005;62:409-416.

5.   Perlis RH, Nierenberg AA, Alpert JE, et al. Effects of adding cognitive therapy to fluoxetine dose increase on risk of relapse and residual depressive symptoms in continuation treatment of major depressive disorder. *J Clin Psychopharmacol.* 2002;22:474-480.

6.   Hensley PL, Nadiga D, Uhlenhuth EH. Long-term effectiveness of cognitive therapy in major depressive disorder. *Depress Anxiety.* 2004;20:1-7.

7.   Hollon SD, DeRubeis RJ, Shelton RC, et al. Prevention of relapse following cognitive therapy vs medications in moderate to severe depression. *Arch Gen Psychiatry.* 2005;62:417-422.

8.   Paykel ES, Scott J, Cornwall PL, et al. Duration of relapse prevention after cognitive therapy in residual depression: follow-up of controlled trial. *Psychol Med.* 2005;35:59-68.

9.   Fava GA, Ruini C, Rafanelli C, Finos L, Conti S, Grandi S. Six-year outcome of cognitive behavior therapy for prevention of recurrent depression. *Am J Psychiatry.* 2004;161:1872-1876.

10.   Swartz HA, Frank E, Shear MK, Thase ME, Fleming MA, Scott J. A pilot study of brief interpersonal psychotherapy for depression among women. *Psychiatr Serv.* 2004;55:448-450.

11.   Frank E, Grochocinski VJ, Spanier CA, et al. Interpersonal psychotherapy and antidepressant medication: evaluation of a sequential treatment strategy in women with recurrent major depression. *J Clin Psychiatry.* 2000;61:51-57.

12.   Browne G, Steiner M, Roberts J, et al. Sertraline and/or interpersonal psychotherapy for patients with dysthymic disorder in primary care: 6-month comparison with longitudinal 2-year follow-up of effectiveness and costs. *J Affect Disord.* 2002;68:317-330.

13.   Harkness KL, Frank E, Anderson B, Houck PR, Luther J, Kupfer DJ. Does interpersonal psychotherapy protect women from depression in the face of stressful life events? *J Consult Clin Psychol.* 2002;70:908-915.

14.   Frank E, Kupfer DJ, Buysse DJ, et al. Randomized trial of weekly, twice-monthly, and monthly interpersonal psychotherapy as maintenance treatment for women with recurrent depression. *Am J Psychiatry.* 2007;164:761-767.

15.   Dowrick C, Dunn G, Ayuso-Mateos JL, et al. Problem solving treatment and group psychoeducation for depression: multicentre randomised controlled trial. Outcomes of Depression International Network (ODIN) Group. *BMJ.* 2000;321:1450-1454.

16.   Mynors-Wallis LM, Gath DH, Day A, Baker F. Randomised controlled trial of problem solving treatment, antidepressant medication, and combined treatment for major depression in primary care. *BMJ.* 2000;320:26-30.

17.   Pampallona S, Bollini P, Tibaldi G, Kupelnick B, Munizza C. Combined pharmacotherapy and psychological treatment for depression: a systematic review. *Arch Gen Psychiatry.* 2004;61:714-719.

18.   Simon J, Pilling S, Burbeck R, Goldberg D. Treatment options in moderate and severe depression: decision analysis supporting a clinical guideline. *Br J Psychiatry.* 2006;189:494-501.

19.   de Maat SM, Dekker J, Schoevers RA, de Jonghe F. Relative efficacy of psychotherapy and combined therapy in the treatment of depression: a meta-analysis. *Eur Psychiatry.* 2007;22:1-8.

20.   Arnow BA, Constantino MJ. Effectiveness of psychotherapy and combination treatment for chronic depression. *J Clin Psychol.* 2003;59:893-905.

21.   Nemeroff CB, Heim CM, Thase ME, et al. Differential responses to psychotherapy versus pharmacotherapy in patients with chronic forms of major depression and childhood trauma. *Proc Natl Acad Sci U S A.* 2003;100:14293-14296.

22.   Kool S, Dekker J, Duijsens IJ, de Jonghe F, Puite B. Efficacy of combined therapy and pharmacotherapy for depressed patients with or without personality disorders. *Harv Rev Psychiatry.* 2003;11:133-141.

23.   Reynolds CF, 3rd, Frank E, Perel JM, et al. Nortriptyline and interpersonal psychotherapy as maintenance therapies for recurrent major depression: a randomized controlled trial in patients older than 59 years. *JAMA.* 1999;281:39-45.

24.   Fink M, Taylor MA. Electroconvulsive therapy: evidence and challenges. *JAMA.* 2007;298:330-332.

25.   Greenberg RM, Kellner CH. Electroconvulsive therapy: a selected review. *Am J Geriatr Psychiatry.* 2005;13:268-281.

26.   Kho KH, van Vreeswijk MF, Simpson S, Zwinderman AH. A meta-analysis of electroconvulsive therapy efficacy in depression. *J ECT.* 2003;19:139-147.

27.   Efficacy and safety of electroconvulsive therapy in depressive disorders: a systematic review and meta-analysis. *Lancet.* 2003;361:799-808.

28.   Fochtmann LJ, Gelenberg AJ. Guideline Watch: Practice Guideline for the Treatment of Patients With Major Depressive Disorder. 2005. http://www.psych.org/psych_pract/treatg/pg/prac_guide.cfm. Published Last Modified Date[. Accessed Dated Accessed].

29.   Husain MM, Rush AJ, Fink M, et al. Speed of response and remission in major depressive disorder with acute electroconvulsive therapy (ECT): a Consortium for Research in ECT (CORE) report. *J Clin Psychiatry.* 2004;65:485-491.

30.   Kellner CH, Knapp RG, Petrides G, et al. Continuation electroconvulsive therapy vs pharmacotherapy for relapse prevention in major depression: a multisite study from the Consortium for Research in Electroconvulsive Therapy (CORE). *Arch Gen Psychiatry.* 2006;63:1337-1344.

31.   Sackeim HA, Haskett RF, Mulsant BH, et al. Continuation pharmacotherapy in the prevention of relapse following electroconvulsive therapy: a randomized controlled trial. *JAMA.* 2001;285:1299-1307.

32.   Marano CM, Phatak P, Vemulapalli UR, et al. Increased plasma concentration of brain-derived neurotrophic factor with electroconvulsive therapy: a pilot study in patients with major depression. *J Clin Psychiatry.* 2007;68:512-517.

33.   Nemeroff CB, Mayberg HS, Krahl SE, et al. VNS therapy in treatment-resistant depression: clinical evidence and putative neurobiological mechanisms. *Neuropsychopharmacology.* 2006;31:1345-1355.

34.   Rush AJ, Marangell LB, Sackeim HA, et al. Vagus nerve stimulation for treatment-resistant depression: a randomized, controlled acute phase trial. *Biol Psychiatry.* 2005;58:347-354.

35.   Rush AJ, Sackeim HA, Marangell LB, et al. Effects of 12 months of vagus nerve stimulation in treatment-resistant depression: a naturalistic study. *Biol Psychiatry.* 2005;58:355-363.

36.   George MS, Rush AJ, Marangell LB, et al. A one-year comparison of vagus nerve stimulation with treatment as usual for treatment-resistant depression. *Biol Psychiatry.* 2005;58:364-373.

37.   Rossini PM, Rossi S. Transcranial magnetic stimulation: diagnostic, therapeutic, and research potential. *Neurology.* 2007;68:484-488.

38.   Kluger BM, Triggs WJ. Use of transcranial magnetic stimulation to influence behavior. *Curr Neurol Neurosci Rep.* 2007;7:491-497.

39.   Eranti S, Mogg A, Pluck G, et al. A randomized, controlled trial with 6-month follow-up of repetitive transcranial magnetic stimulation and electroconvulsive therapy for severe depression. *Am J Psychiatry.* 2007;164:73-81.

40.   Loo CK, Mitchell PB, McFarquhar TF, Malhi GS, Sachdev PS. A sham-controlled trial of the efficacy and safety of twice-daily rTMS in major depression. *Psychol Med.* 2007;37:341-349.

41. Mogg A, Pluck G, Eranti SV, et al. A randomized controlled trial with 4-month follow-up of adjunctive repetitive transcranial magnetic stimulation of the left prefrontal cortex for depression. *Psychol Med.* 2007:1-11.

42. Couturier JL. Efficacy of rapid-rate repetitive transcranial magnetic stimulation in the treatment of depression: a systematic review and meta-analysis. *J Psychiatry Neurosci.* 2005;30:83-90.

43. Herrmann LL, Ebmeier KP. Factors modifying the efficacy of transcranial magnetic stimulation in the treatment of depression: a review. *J Clin Psychiatry.* 2006;67:1870-1876.

44. Brunelin J, Poulet E, Boeuve C, Zeroug-vial H, d'Amato T, Saoud M. [Efficacy of repetitive transcranial magnetic stimulation (rTMS) in major depression: a review]. *Encephale.* 2007;33:126-134.

45. Kosel M, Frick C, Lisanby SH, Fisch HU, Schlaepfer TE. Magnetic seizure therapy improves mood in refractory major depression. *Neuropsychopharmacology.* 2003;28:2045-2048.

46. Lisanby SH, Luber B, Schlaepfer TE, Sackeim HA. Safety and feasibility of magnetic seizure therapy (MST) in major depression: randomized within-subject comparison with electroconvulsive therapy. *Neuropsychopharmacology.* 2003;28:1852-1865.

47. White PF, Amos Q, Zhang Y, et al. Anesthetic considerations for magnetic seizure therapy: a novel therapy for severe depression. *Anesth Analg.* 2006;103:76-80, table of contents.

48. Johansen-Berg H, Gutman DA, Behrens TE, et al. Anatomical Connectivity of the Subgenual Cingulate Region Targeted with Deep Brain Stimulation for Treatment-Resistant Depression. *Cereb Cortex.* 2007.

49. Mayberg HS, Lozano AM, Voon V, et al. Deep brain stimulation for treatment-resistant depression. *Neuron.* 2005;45:651-660.

50. Gregoire AJ, Kumar R, Everitt B, Henderson AF, Studd JW. Transdermal oestrogen for treatment of severe postnatal depression. *Lancet.* 1996;347:930-933.

51. Smith RN, Studd JW, Zamblera D, Holland EF. A randomised comparison over 8 months of 100 micrograms and 200 micrograms twice weekly doses of transdermal oestradiol in the treatment of severe premenstrual syndrome. *Br J Obstet Gynaecol.* 1995;102:475-484.

52. Soares CN, Almeida OP, Joffe H, Cohen LS. Efficacy of estradiol for the treatment of depressive disorders in perimenopausal women: a double-blind, randomized, placebo-controlled trial. *Arch Gen Psychiatry.* 2001;58:529-534.

53. Rutledge R, Dorghazi P, Peralgie C. Efficacy of estradiol topical patch in the treatment of symptoms of depression following mini-gastric bypass in women. *Obes Surg.* 2006;16:1221-1226.

54. Stahl SM, Grady MM. Differences in mechanism of action between current and future antidepressants. *J Clin Psychiatry.* 2003;64 Suppl 13:13-17.

55. Rediger JD, Summers L. Mindfulness training and meditation. In: Lake J, Spiegel D, eds. *Complementary and Alternative Treatments in Mental Health Care.* Arlington, VA: American Psychiatric Publishing, Inc.; 2006.

56. Coelho HF, Canter PH, Ernst E. Mindfulness-based cognitive therapy: evaluating current evidence and informing future research. *J Consult Clin Psychol.* 2007;75:1000-1005.

57. Zhang GJ, Shi ZY, Liu S, Gong SH, Liu JQ, Liu JS. Clinical observation on treatment of depression by electro-acupuncture combined with Paroxetine. *Chin J Integr Med.* 2007;13:228-230.

58. Quah-Smith JI, Tang WM, Russell J. Laser acupuncture for mild to moderate depression in a primary care setting--a randomised controlled trial. *Acupunct Med.* 2005;23:103-111.

59. Gallagher SM, Allen JJ, Hitt SK, Schnyer RN, Manber R. Six-month depression relapse rates among women treated with acupuncture. *Complement Ther Med.* 2001;9:216-218.

60. Allen JJ, Schnyer RN, Chambers AS, Hitt SK, Moreno FA, Manber R. Acupuncture for depression: a randomized controlled trial. *J Clin Psychiatry.* 2006;67:1665-1673.

61. Even C, Schroder CM, Friedman S, Rouillon F. Efficacy of light therapy in nonseasonal depression: A systematic review. *J Affect Disord.* 2007.

62. Terman M, Terman JS. Light therapy for seasonal and nonseasonal depression: efficacy, protocol, safety, and side effects. *CNS Spectr.* 2005;10:647-663; quiz 672.

63. Tuunainen A, Kripke DF, Endo T. Light therapy for non-seasonal depression. *Cochrane Database Syst Rev.* 2004:CD004050.

64. Krishnamurthy MN, Telles S. Assessing depression following two ancient Indian interventions: effects of yoga and ayurveda on older adults in a residential home. *J Gerontol Nurs.* 2007;33:17-23.

65. Plotkin BJ, Rodos JJ, Kappler R, et al. Adjunctive osteopathic manipulative treatment in women with depression: a pilot study. *J Am Osteopath Assoc.* 2001;101:517-523.

66. Wilkinson SM, Love SB, Westcombe AM, et al. Effectiveness of aromatherapy massage in the management of anxiety and depression in patients with cancer: a multicenter randomized controlled trial. *J Clin Oncol.* 2007;25:532-539.

Chapter 6

Mechanisms and Interconnections within the Functional Medicine Matrix Model

As documented in preceding chapters, there is an urgent need for an approach to treating depression that goes beyond that of conventional pharmaceutical, psychological, and other types of interventions. The prevailing conventional paradigm focuses exclusively on dysregulation in neurophysiology and psychosocial function. While clearly important, there are many other influences on depression that are usually not assessed or are given only passing notice in the conventional model. In this chapter, we will examine the scientific research on dysregulation in a variety of areas. In functional medicine, we view these diverse influences through a prism called the *Functional Medicine Matrix Model* (see Figure 6.1). Evaluating these core systems helps to uncover a rich collection of underlying antecedents, triggers, and mediators that may be linked to depression. Remediating underlying dysfunction is likely to have a highly beneficial effect on many patients with depressive disorders, resulting in improved outcomes for a greater number of people.

Hormone and Neurotransmitter Regulation

Hormonal imbalances are particularly relevant to the discussion of depression. There is a wealth of information implicating the stress response and hypothalamic-pituitary-adrenal (HPA) axis imbalances as triggers and mediators of depression. The research literature shows connections between depression and cortisol, thyroid, melatonin, insulin, estradiol, testosterone, and various brain neurotransmitters.

The Stress Response System and Depression

The stress response system (SRS) is the major neurophysiological basis of the mind-body connection. Stress responses and depression share many common signs, symptoms, mediators, and neural pathways. They are not synonymous, nor can depression be conceptualized solely as a dysregulation of the SRS. Nevertheless, understanding the dysregulation that occurs within the SRS is critical to an appreciation of the varying manifestations of depression and to integrating the expanded paradigm advanced in this monograph.

Depressogenic factors may originate within the body (e.g., Addison's disease, a pituitary microadenoma), the psyche (e.g., faulty cognitions or attributions), and the environment (e.g., a failing marriage, exposure to abuse, loss of a parent, unemployment). Genetic predispositions from first-degree relatives also play a role. However, regardless of the point or points of origin, depressogenic factors are transduced bidirectionally via the SRS into morphological and functional changes within both the brain and peripheral target tissues (e.g., cardiovascular, gonadal, immune, musculoskeletal).

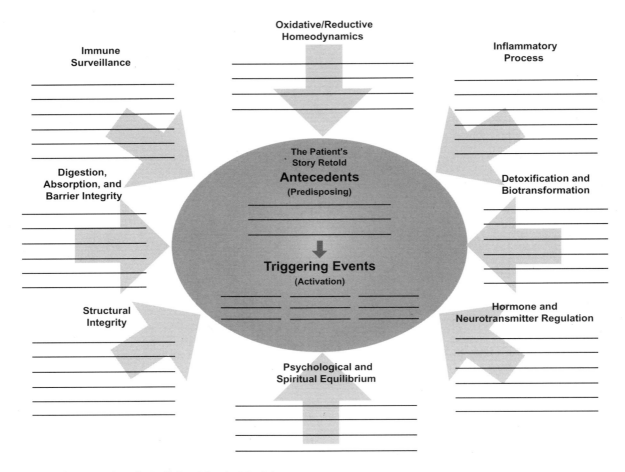

Figure 6.1—The Functional Medicine Matrix Model

©2007, The Institute for Functional Medicine

The SRS can be divided into both a core and a secondary aspect. The core parts of the SRS include the HPA axis and the locus ceruleus (LC). The LC is a nucleus of cells that contains virtually all of the norepinephrine-containing neurons in the brain. A single LC neuron can terminate on over 100,000 other neurons, so one can imagine the far-ranging effects of this small mid-pons nucleus. Under normal conditions, the LC helps maintain alertness. The secondary SRS includes the prefrontal cortex (PFC), the amygdala, and the hippocampus.[1]

Primary mediators of the stress response include neuropeptides (corticotropin-releasing hormone [CRH], arginine vasopressin [AVP], adrenocorticotrophic hormone [ACTH]), neurotransmitters (norepinephrine, epinephrine, serotonin, glutamate, acetylcholine), and the well-known stress hormone cortisol.

Primary triggers of the stress response may be physiological (inflammation, extremes of temperature, pain, hypoglycemia, hypovolemia, excess exercise) and act directly via activation of the LC, or they may be perceptual/experiential (unbidden novelty, unpredictability, trauma, loss of control over self and self-concept) and act via the secondary SRS.

The Acute Stress Response

Under acute conditions of actual or perceived stress, the SRS promotes rapid, instinctual, stereotypical behaviors that generally fall into the fight-or-flight category. In potentially stressful situations, the amygdala receives sensory

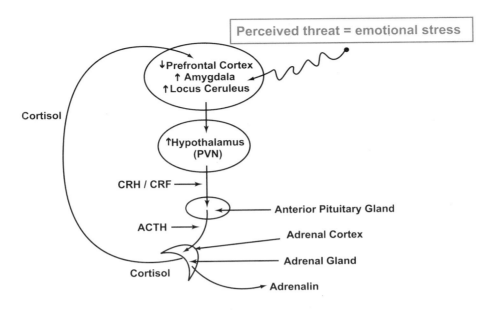

Figure 6.2—The HPA Axis and Hormonal Cascade in the Stress Response

input, assigns an experientially based valence (safe, arousing, or dangerous) to situations, and only then sends information to the PFC. Because of this, we often experience instantaneous gut reactions to people and events for reasons we cannot consciously explain.

Once activated, the acute stress response is manifested by both a peripheral mobilization (sympathetic activation of the autonomic nervous system) and a central change in brain function favoring an inhibition of PFC higher-order thinking and an activation of limbic and brain stem structures. This is experienced as anxiety, panic, activation, or even terrifying paralysis, all accompanied by an inability to think in an objective, thoughtful, and analytical manner (impaired executive functions of judgment, organization, planning, working memory). The stress response affects critical vegetative functions—alertness, appetite, metabolic activity, and autonomic, reproductive, neuroendocrine, immune, gastrointestinal, and psychomotor functions are all disrupted in a reverberating, bidirectional manner within the depressive experience. *This linkage is one of the facts supporting a functional medicine approach to depressive disorders.*

Neurophysiologically, the acute stress response is activated when the amygdala, drawing on conditioned memory stored in other parts of the brain, including the hippocampus and striatum, receives sensory input that associates an experience with danger (based on past experience). Projections from the amygdala to the norepinephrine-containing neurons of the LC are activated. The LC then transmits a norepinephrine "alarm" via its projections throughout the brain and periphery. LC projections include those to:

- The dorsolateral PFC (inhibiting its executive, higher-order thinking function)
- The lower brain stem (including serotonergic raphe nuclei and the solitary nucleus associated with anxiety)
- The autonomic nervous system (which activates the sympathetic and inhibits the parasympathetic physiology)
- The hypothalamus (which then releases CRH, AVP, and downstream ACTH and cortisol)
- The amygdala itself

The amygdala, activated by this positive feedback loop mediated by norepinephrine, CRH, AVP, and cortisol, releases its own stores of CRH to continue the feedback loop. Once the stressor has been removed, the system reestablishes homeostasis; however, key elements of the situation have been stored (by the amygdala, hippocampus, and striatum) for future reference.[2]

> **Clinical Pearl:**
>
> I recently noted the lingering effects of the acute stress response in a patient who had depression accompanied by an attachment problem. Her mother's affect was always extreme and unpredictable, invoking repeated fear/danger responses in the patient. When the patient came in for a visit after an extended absence, she was highly anxious because she didn't know how I was going to behave. This anxiety made it quite difficult for her to direct the conversation in any meaningful way. She calmed down immediately when I identified the fear and gave her information about what I was doing. Within seconds of knowing that she was not in danger from me, she began to direct the conversation to her real concerns.

The Chronic Stress Response in Depression

The physiological wear and tear that the body experiences due to repeated cycles of stress, during which it attempts to maintain stability via continuous rebalancing, has been termed allostasis (maintaining stability or homeostasis through change).[3] Allostatic load is the cumulative physiological strain that is required to maintain homeostasis.[4] Markers of allostatic load are being refined and tested. At the current time, they are thought to include 10 variables, six of which seem to be related to metabolic syndrome (HgA1c, waist-hip ratio, HDL, total cholesterol, systolic and diastolic blood pressure) and four of which are related to the HPA axis (urinary epinephrine, norepinephrine, cortisol, DHEA-S).[5] Cumulative measures of allostatic load are a significant predictor of all-cause mortality, cognitive decline, physical functioning, and cardiovascular disease for as long as 7.5 years after initial measurement. (For an overview of the effects of acute and chronic stress, both psychological and physical, see Tatum[6] in the *Textbook of Functional Medicine*.)

Depression exhibits characteristics of a *chronically* activated SRS, resulting in an increased allostatic load. The mediators and consequences of chronic stress have all been associated, in one way or another, with depression. As described above, the primary mediators of the stress response include CRH, AVP, ACTH, cortisol, DHEA, DHEA-S, norepinephrine, and epinephrine. Secondary pathways include cellular responses such as second and third messenger activation, enzymatic activation, receptor modulation, short- and long-term potentiation, apoptosis, and changes in neurotrophic factors, glial cell function, and immune parameters including cytokines. At a tertiary level, these processes are evident in altered markers that reflect a summation and integration of the secondary processes, such as blood pressure, heart rate, and HgA1C. At the quaternary level are diagnosable diseases (e.g., heart diseases, diabetes, cognitive impairment).

The onset of depression may be due to many factors, including:

- The persistence of a chronic and real stressor (e.g., a state of externally induced helplessness over one's career or finances due to illness; war; in a child, an abusive or abandoning parent)
- The triggering of a biological or genetic program (e.g., a severe inflammatory disorder or a strongly heritable disorder)
- A failure to realign one's beliefs or actions as part of an adaptive response to a life situation (e.g., giving up an idealized view of marriage)
- A skill deficit (e.g., a child with an unrecognized learning disability who is trying to achieve normally)

Regardless of cause, however, the SRS seems to become and remain dysregulated as part of the genesis and maintenance of the depressive condition.[7] In the midst of this chronic activation, the depression is transduced into physical manifestations that are the basis for the comorbidity associated with depression.

Cortisol and Adrenal Fatigue

The HPA axis has major interactions with the hypothalamic-pituitary-gonadal (HPG) and reproductive hormone axes, the thyroid axis, the growth hormone axis, glucoregulation, insulin resistance, and Th1/Th2 balance. Abnormalities of all these perpetuate the cycle of depression.[8] For example, a person who is repeatedly hypoglycemic (perhaps due to poor diet, chromium deficiency, or high levels of stress and pain) will, over time, stress the adrenal axis. The stress response is quite complex and the levels of cortisol, DHEA, other adrenal steroids, and catecholamines vary with the duration of the stress, genetic factors, and the consequent phase of adrenal insufficiency or overstimulation. Depending on the duration of the stresses, genetic factors, early life experiences, and factors affecting resilience (e.g., social support), the pattern and severity of adrenal axis dysfunction, as seen on the salivary adrenal index and measures of catecholamine turnover (e.g., 24-hour urinary catecholamines), will differ.[9] Early in the stress response (in this example, it is secondary to hypoglycemia), one might see elevated cortisol and catecholamines, but with time (months or years of repeated and frequent hypoglycemic episodes), poor nutrition, and continued stressors, the system's ability to produce cortisol, DHEA, and other adrenal steroids may be reduced and reserves of catecholamines depleted, leaving the patient fatigued, exhausted, and unable to mount an adequate stress response on an hour-to-hour and situation to situation basis. This can easily present to the clinician as depression. Some studies, but not all, support the efficacy of DHEA use in depression, often with supraphysiological doses.[10, 11]

Thyroid Dysfunction

The thyroid axis is closely aligned with central beta-receptor function, DNA expression of neurotrophic factors, serotonergic and noradrenergic receptor function,[12] and melatonin. This alignment is thought to underlie the finding that although the vast majority of patients with major depression are euthyroid, the condition often coexists with autoimmune subclinical thyroiditis, suggesting that depression may alter the immune system or that it may be an autoimmune disorder itself.[13] According to a 2006 review article, "It is clear that depression is not characterized by an overt thyroid dysfunction, but it is also clear that a subgroup of depressed patients may manifest subtle thyroid abnormalities, or an activation of an autoimmune process."[13] Evidence of causality is conflicting, since changes in the hypothalamic-pituitary-thyroid (HPT) axis could be either causes or consequences of affective disorders; in addition, the cause could be thyroid peroxidase antibodies and not thyroid hormone levels, per se.

Recent evidence of thyroid dysfunction in depression includes the following:

- A prospective cohort study found that patients hospitalized with hypothyroidism had a greater risk of readmission with depression or bipolar disorder than control patients hospitalized with either osteoarthritis or nontoxic goiter.[14]
- 23% of 60 depressed patients with "high-normal" (3.00–5.50 mIU/L) TSH levels had an exaggerated TSH response on the thyrotropin-releasing hormone stimulation test. This prevalence was significantly greater than the 6% prevalence of positive stimulation test results reported in the euthyroid general population.[15]
- In a population of chronically depressed patients referred to a mood disorders unit, 22% of those referred with treatment-resistant depression had evidence of clinical or subclinical hypothyroidism compared with 2% of those with non-treatment-resistant depression.[16]
- Mean antenatal T4 concentrations and free T4 indices correlated significantly and negatively with mean depression scores during each of 3 postpartum time periods.[17]
- Subjects with at least one diagnosis of anxiety or mood disorders were positive for serum antithyroid peroxidase more frequently than subjects without mood or anxiety disorders.[18]

T3 therapy has been shown to improve patient response when used to augment antidepressants in treatment-resistant depression.[19, 20] (See *Strategies for Enhancing Antidepressant Effectiveness* in Chapter 4.) A 2006 review[12] described a possible mechanism: administration of a combination of fluoxetine and T3 induced reductions in the transcription of the 5-HT1A and 5-HT1B autoreceptors, which mediate serotonergic neurotransmission by feedback actions at the levels of cell firing and neurotransmitter release. It has been suggested that T3 may be beneficial in approximately 25% of depressed patients.[21]

There is also evidence showing the effectiveness of T4 as an antidepressant augmentation strategy.[22] A 2000 review of 8 open clinical trials reported: "Augmentation with supraphysiological doses of T4 has antidepressant and prophylactic effects in roughly 50% of patients completely resistant to all other antidepressant and prophylactic therapies.... It has also consistently been shown that high serum concentrations of T4 predict favorable response to antidepressant treatment and that the serum levels of T4 decrease in responders to these treatments, but not in non-responders."[23]

Circadian Rhythm and Melatonin

Evidence for a dysfunction in circadian time keeping in depression includes the cyclic nature of depressive illness, the diurnal variations in its symptomatology, and the existence of disturbed sleep-wake and core body temperature rhythms. Thus, the rhythm regulator melatonin has received attention as a marker of mood disorders. "Measurement of melatonin either in saliva or plasma, or of its main metabolite 6-sulfatoxymelatonin in urine, have documented significant alterations in melatonin secretion in depressive patients during the acute phase of illness. Both the levels and the timing of melatonin secretion are altered in bipolar affective disorder and in patients with seasonal affective disorder (SAD)."[24] While melatonin treatment has been shown effective in treating circadian rhythm disorders as well as insomnia, the inference that it would also influence affective disorders has not been completely borne out.[25] However, bright light treatment that suppresses melatonin production is effective in treating bipolar affective disorder and SAD, winter type,[24] and this intervention also showed some clinical response in non-seasonal depression in a randomized controlled trial (RCT).[26]

New avenues for treatment in this area have focused on compounds with activity at melatonergic receptors. In several clinical trials, agomelatine, a compound with agonistic properties at MT1 and MT2 receptors and antagonistic properties at the 5-HT2C receptor, has been found superior to placebo, with suggested superior efficacy to currently available antidepressants. The rate of effect and overall tolerability profile of agomelatine also suggests a clinical advantage over selective serotonin reuptake inhibitors (SSRIs) and serotonin/norepinephrine reuptake inhibitors (SNRIs).[27] For a larger discussion, see a review[25] of the antidepressant mechanisms of agomelatine, as well as studies of melatonin in depression.

Reproductive Hormones

Estradiol, testosterone, and other reproductive hormones interact with brain neurotransmitters.[28-30] In particular, altered levels of estrogens can have mood-altering effects for many different reasons. These alterations are thought to occur via direct estrogen effects on cell surface receptors or gene expression (e.g., altered genetic dendritic formation in the hippocampus during different phases of the menstrual cycle)[31] or via increased or decreased availability of catecholamines due to competition for catechol-O-methyltransferase (COMT); this competition for COMT is especially significant in individuals with reduced COMT enzymatic activity due to single nucleotide polymorphisms (SNPs) or undermethylation.[32] Recent research has indicated that estradiol impacts CRH gene expression.[33] This suggests a link between estrogen and the HPA axis, which is so central to the biological aspects of depression.

The intricate association between the HPG and HPA axes (the HPA axis directly inhibits gonadotropin-releasing hormone) is exemplified by increasing rates of depression in women of reproductive age; by increased risk of depression for women who are perimenopausal or postmenopausal or in the postpartum stage; and by the responsiveness of perimenopausal and menopausal depression,[34-36] premenstrual depression,[37] and postnatal depression[38] to transdermal estrogen.[39] For postmenopausal women, however, hormone replacement therapy (estrogen plus proges-terone or estrogen alone) was no more effective than placebo in some studies.[40-42]

Approximately 20% of men in their 60s and 50% of men over the age of 80 demonstrate low testosterone levels. This age-associated hypogonadism is associated with some symptoms that overlap with depression, but the exact association is unclear. Two recent studies have found that low testosterone levels predicted earlier onset and greater incidence of depressive illness,[43, 44] but studies of testosterone replacement in depressed men were conflicting.[45-50] Similarly, it has been proposed that replacement of DHEA may improve mood and libido in both men and women. Although there is some limited evidence of mood-enhancing effects of DHEA,[51] particularly in populations with adrenal insufficiency,[52, 53] the literature does not currently support its therapeutic use in this area, and more defined and specific clinical trials are needed.[54] In addition, risks of long-term supplementation with either testosterone or DHEA are unknown.

Glucoregulation

The association between affective disorders and alterations in glucose utilization is well established. (See Chapter 3 for a discussion of diabetes and depression.) Depressed patients demonstrate significantly higher basal glucose lev-els, greater cumulative glucose responses after an oral glucose tolerance test, and larger cumulative insulin responses after an oral glucose tolerance test than control subjects, indicating a functional state of insulin resistance during major depressive illness.[55] While several studies found that the severity of depressive symptoms increased the risk for insulin resistance,[56-59] other research was contradictory.[60, 61] In a 2006 study, insulin sensitivity increased in nondia-betic patients after successful treatment with an SSRI or a tricyclic antidepressant (TCA).[62] A possible explanation for insulin resistance in depressive disorders (and Alzheimer's disease) holds that inadequate glucose utilization underlies neuronal changes in crucial brain regions (i.e., the limbic system), and in patients with undetected or untreated insu-lin resistance, such changes in glucose utilization may lead to neurodegeneration.[63] A 2002 review[64] postulated that insulin resistance may be the link between depression and atherosclerotic vascular diseases.

Immune Surveillance

Immune system dysfunction and dysregulation—with or without an inflammatory association—have significant relationships with depression. Supporting the concepts advanced in this monograph, there is recent and mounting evidence that both glial cells (as active participants in synaptic transmission, supporters of neuronal function, clear-ance agents for neurotransmitters such as glutamate from the synapse, and modulators of synaptic plasticity) and glutamate[65, 66] are involved in depressive disorders[67] and that the immune system is disturbed both peripherally and centrally in depression. At least one recent study reported a response to riluzole augmentation for patients with treat-ment-resistant depression; riluzole targets glutamate neurotransmission.[68]

Additionally, lamotrigine, a glutamate inhibitor,[69] has recently been documented to have antidepressant ef-fects in unipolar depression in 2 small studies.[70, 71] While the specific pathways by which glutamate and glia influ-ence mood disorders are not fully understood,[72] current thought indicates that activation of the proinflammatory cytokines activates the tryptophan- and serotonin-degrading enzyme system indoleamine 2,3-dioxygenase (IDO), which may contribute to the serotonergic dysregulation in depression. IDO and its subsequent enzyme kynurenine monooxygenase increase production of quinolinic acid, a strong agonist of the ionotropic (fast-acting) glutamater-gic N-methyl-D-aspartate (NMDA) receptor.[73] Glutamatergic overactivity is generally thought to be neurotoxic via calcium-mediated apoptotic pathways. In addition, the metabotropic glutamatergic receptors (involved in the long-term modulation of glutamate transmission) can facilitate the release of serotonin, norepinephrine, and dopamine.[74] This imbalance in glutamate activity is normally counteracted by a subset of glia, the astrocytes, whose numbers are reduced in depression.[75] Thus, imbalances in the immune-neurotransmitter systems are likely to form part of the genesis or maintenance of some forms of depression.

Another line of evidence supporting the role of the immune system in mood disorders stems from the fact that several illnesses characterized by disturbances in the immune system (e.g., lupus, rheumatoid arthritis, celiac disease) are often accompanied by depression, as discussed in Chapter 3. While hypotheses regarding the connection between psychiatric symptoms and autoimmune abnormalities have yet to be proved, there is strong evidence that the same alterations in immunity may play a role in the pathophysiology of both depressive symptoms and these inflammatory disorders. A 2006 review[76] summarizing the evidence for a cytokine-mediated pathogenesis of depression and fatigue in multiple sclerosis reported that peripheral and central production of cytokines may account for some of the behavioral symptoms that cannot be explained by psychosocial factors or central nervous system (CNS) damage. In fact, emerging clinical data from multiple sclerosis patients support an association of central inflammation, as measured by MRI, and inflammatory markers with depressive symptoms and fatigue.

Does delayed food sensitivity (i.e., IgG food allergy) result in an IgG immune complex-induced activation of inflammation? Could this contribute to depression? When one begins to appreciate the link between the immune system, the HPA axis, and the endocrine system, the possibility that food and mood are linked via an immune response to food (the intestines contain nearly 70% of the body's immune cells[77]) becomes plausible. Recent research using the 2002 Canadian Community Health Study confirmed an association between allergies and mood and anxiety disorders in a general population sample.[78]

Inflammatory Process

Immunologically, central CRH inhibits inflammation via glucocorticoids and catecholamines, but immune CRH stimulates inflammation. Numerous inflammatory abnormalities have been associated with depression,[79-82] including changes in acute-phase proteins and cytokines. These products of immune activation are known to have direct effects on the HPA axis, the sympathetic nervous system, energy balance, and neuronal function.

The *cytokine hypothesis of depression*[83] suggests that the nervous system, the endocrine system, and the immune system are reciprocally linked as both triggering and mediating pathways of depression. In this view, a variety of proinflammatory cytokines (IL-1, IL-6, TNF-alpha, gamma interferon) act as neuromodulating mediators affecting behavioral, neurochemical, and endocrine features of depressive disorders. The cytokines are thought to account for the HPA overactivity characteristic of melancholic depression, since cytokines are known to cross and influence the blood-brain barrier (if produced peripherally) and to disturb the negative feedback inhibition of corticosteroids in the HPA axis. Major bodies of evidence supporting this aspect of depression include:

- A significantly increased risk for suicide has been associated with asthma[84] and seasonal allergy.[85]
- In a recent national epidemiological study in the United States, a doubling of the rate of suicide in women during periods of highest pollen counts was demonstrated, after adjustment for environmental light.[86]
- In a double-blind, crossover study involving 20 healthy males without a history of psychiatric disorder, subthreshold doses of non-infectious endotoxin induced elevation of specific cytokines, including TNF-alpha and IL-6, associated with significantly increased anxiety, impaired memory, and depressed mood.[87]

According to Dantzer, it is possible to describe a very close connection between inflammation, illness, and depression:

"In response to a peripheral infection, innate immune cells produce pro-inflammatory cytokines that act on the brain to cause sickness behaviour. When activation of the peripheral immune system continues unabated, such as during systemic infections, cancer or autoimmune diseases, the ensuing immune signalling to the brain can lead to an exacerbation of sickness and the development of symptoms of depression in vulnerable individuals. These phenomena might account for the increased prevalence of clinical depression in physically ill people. Inflammation is therefore an important biological event that might increase the risk of major depressive episodes, much like the more traditional psychosocial factors." [88]

Interestingly, in a 2005 study, IL-6 levels were significantly lower after treatment with SSRIs in both patients with major depressive disorder and healthy controls.[89] In a 2007 study, depressed patients who did not respond to SSRIs had significantly higher levels of IL-6 and TNF-alpha than both euthymic patients who were formerly SSRI resistant and healthy controls.

Subtle inflammatory signals that have been shown to be factors in cardiac pathology have also been associated with depression.[90] Several studies have shown that acute-phase proteins including high-sensitivity C-reactive protein and amyloid-A increase in depression.[91-93] The acute-phase response begins with the release of proinflammatory cytokines IL-1 and TNF, which stimulate the release of copious amounts of IL-6 by peripheral cells, including vascular smooth muscle. In response to IL-6, the liver shifts from the synthesis of "housekeeping" proteins such as albumen toward production of acute-phase reactants, which are thought to play a key role in cardiovascular diseases.[94]

The rise in markers of stress and inflammation that occurs in depression also underscores the link between affective illness and metabolic syndrome. A 2007 study was the first to demonstrate that depressive symptoms, stressful life events, and frequent feelings of intense anger and tension predicted the risk for developing metabolic syndrome, as defined by multiple definitions.[95] The authors noted that psychosocial factors are associated with alterations in the autonomic nervous system (e.g., elevated heart rate and reduced heart rate variability), the HPA system (e.g., elevated cortisol), and hemostatic and inflammatory markers (e.g., heightened platelet aggregation, fibrinogen, proinflammatory cytokines, white blood cell count). "All of these physiological changes have been recognized as important in the development of the metabolic syndrome."

Another emerging pathway between depression and inflammation involves melanocyte-stimulating hormone (MSH). According to Lipton, "Alpha-MSH modulates all forms of inflammation by acting on peripheral inflammatory cells, [central] glial inflammatory cells, and on CNS receptors that activate descending anti-inflammatory neural pathways."[96] MSH interacts with the nearby melatonin receptor to regulate restorative, restful sleep. MSH is made by cleavage of a parent molecule, proopiomelanocortin (POMC), following activation of the long isoform of the leptin receptor, a cytokine receptor. Production of MSH is accompanied by production of beta-endorphin. Deficiency of MSH will result in absence of restorative restful sleep and abnormal perception of pain due to melatonin and endorphin problems, respectively. Many people with MSH deficiency will have cytokine-driven leptin resistance; the adipose tissue-derived hormone leptin acts via its receptor (LRb) in the brain to regulate energy balance and neuroendocrine function (e.g., MSH).

This information supports the use of anti-inflammatory strategies in the treatment of depression, including (as appropriate to the patient) reduction of proinflammatory triggers and their mediators (e.g., identifying food sensitivities and withdrawing offending foods, reducing exposure to respiratory allergens and toxins); treatment of chronic infections; normalization of insulin and glucose regulation; and use of anti-inflammatory compounds such as curcumin (turmeric) or COX-2 inhibitors. Several recent studies on the effects of curcumin in chronically stressed rats have confirmed its antidepressant activity, related to its modulating effects on the HPA axis, hippocampal neurons, and serotonergic receptors.[97-100] Similarly, stressed mice treated with the COX-2 inhibitor celecoxib had lower levels of proinflammatory cytokines than stressed mice who did not receive the treatment,[101] and another experiment suggests additional neuroprotective and antioxidant functions of these medications under stress-induced conditions.[102]

Digestion, Absorption, and Barrier Integrity

The alimentary tract and its accessory organs (liver, gallbladder, and pancreas), the gut-associated lymphoid tissue (GALT), the active microbial populations, and the epithelial barrier that separates the outside environment from the inside all constitute important areas for consideration when looking at patients with depression. Numerous studies using animal models have shown that stress can trigger colonic epithelial barrier dysfunction via effects on mast cells, gamma interferon, and myosin light chain phosphorylation.[103-105] This decrease in gut barrier function in turn leads to excessive uptake of luminal material. Thus, depression can increase vulnerability to intestinal inflammation. Research has shown that the presence of an oral antigen during chronic psychological stress altered the immune response to sensitization and caused subsequent antigen-induced gut pathophysiology in rats.[106] In a separate study on mice, pups separated from their mothers had a more severe colitis than those who were not separated. In addition, antidepressant therapy improved parameters of depressive-like behavior and reduced vulnerability to dextran sulphate colitis.[107] Chronic stress has also been shown to increase bacterial uptake in follicle-associated epithelium.[108] Interestingly, in a study that exposed rats to water-avoidance stress, researchers found that pretreatment with probiotics completely prevented stress-induced bacterial adhesion and translocation of bacteria to mesenteric lymph nodes.[109]

Conversely, it has been hypothesized that digestive imbalances can contribute to affective disorders by causing limited nutrient absorption. For example, aging patients, those with *Helicobacter*-induced chronic gastritis, and those who take H2 receptor antagonists often have low-functioning parietal cells in the stomach, resulting in reduced production of hyperchloric acid (stomach acid). This has multiple consequences, including increased risk of constipation and small intestinal bacterial overgrowth (SIBO). Additionally, absorption of vitamin B12 may be reduced when release of intrinsic factor is impaired.[110] Cater reported that "small intestinal bacterial overgrowth in hypochlorhydria probably leads to putrefactive breakdown of the metabolically useful products of protein digestion, thereby reducing their availability for certain essential pathways. The possible lowering of tryptophan, tyrosine, and phenylalanine in the blood may be a precipitating factor in depression in hypochloric patients."[111]

Indeed, there is evidence that inadequate digestion (or ingestion) of protein can result in dysthymia, resistance to antidepressant treatment, or depressive relapse. Tryptophan depletion induces marked reduction in plasma tryptophan, as well as brain serotonin synthesis and release. Depressive symptoms are common in celiac disease, and at least 2 studies suggest that the cause is impaired availability of tryptophan.[112, 113] In several studies, experimental lowering of serotonin neurotransmission by acute tryptophan depletion induced a transient depressed mood in 50% to 60% of remitted depressed patients treated with an SSRI.[114] (However, in currently depressed patients, tryptophan depletion may augment response to an SSNRI.[115]) In addition, catecholamine depletion via a tyrosine hydroxylase inhibitor reversed the therapeutic effects of norepinephrine reuptake inhibitors (NRIs) but not SSRIs.[116]

Bidirectional communication occurs between the CNS and the enteric nervous system, occurring along what has been termed the gut-brain axis. A 2004 review characterized irritable bowel syndrome (IBS) as a model for these gut-brain interactions: "Various non-site specific neurotransmitters influence gastrointestinal, endocrine and immune function, as well as human behavior and emotional state, depending on their location. The physiology of the digestive tract, the subjective experience of symptom, health behavior, and treatment outcome are strongly affected by psychosocial factors."[117] Psychiatric disorders, especially major depression, anxiety, and somatoform disorders, occur among 20 to 50% of IBS syndrome patients.[118] Our understanding of the role of neurotransmitters in IBS has been strengthened by studies showing that corticotrophin-releasing factor (CRF) plays a major part in stress-related gastrointestinal alterations, and in fact, CRF1 receptors are now being investigated as a therapeutic target for IBS.[119]

Detoxification and Biotransformation

Toxins and their biotransformation constitute an important area in relationship to depression. As will be shown, certain toxic metals can have a subtle yet profound effect on mood. Additionally, biotransformation of drugs and endogenously produced hormones can have an important effect on brain function. Consider that the vast majority of psychotropic medications are metabolized in the liver[120, 121]; steroid hormones (e.g., estrogen, testosterone) known to have an effect on mood disorders are metabolized in the liver[122, 123]; and levels of hormones and drugs can become toxic through hepatic recirculation.[124, 125] Thus, the efficacy with which an individual detoxifies these substances can increase or decrease their effect.

The detoxification systems must rid the body of toxins such as xenobiotics, which can cause neurological damage. For example, lead exposure has been linked with biochemical and functional changes in the heme biosynthetic pathway and in the renal, cardiovascular, endocrine, immune, and nervous systems. As Needleman determined 20 years ago, "Encephalopathy generally occurs at blood lead levels of 80 µg/dL or more, but unequivocal brain damage has been demonstrated at doses well below this level. At lower doses, the neurocognitive effects of lead are expressed as diminished psychometric intelligence, attention deficits, conduct problems, alterations in the electroencephalogram, school failure, and increased referral rates for special needs."[126] In addition to its direct physiological effects, lead is associated with deficiencies in body calcium, zinc, iron, and protein stores. Lead also has been shown to cause increased neuropsychiatric symptoms, including mood disorders, many years after exposure.[127] One psychiatrist has written a personal account of the effects of lead poisoning in his patients.[128] A 2000 study showed a significant dose-response relationship between career solvent exposure, blood lead level, and personality symptoms in journeyman painters. "Results showed that the probability of being diagnosed with a mood disorder differed significantly in painters (41%) and control subjects (16%).... Painters exhibited a sub-clinical pattern of personality dysfunction involving symptomatology that was measured allowing for late onset (after age 25)."[129]

There is also evidence that mercury can induce depression-like behavior. A 2007 review on methylmercury reported: "Several mechanisms have been suggested from in vivo and in vitro studies, such as effects on neurotransmitter systems, induction of oxidative stress and disruption of microtubules and intracellular calcium homeostasis. Recent in vitro data show that very low levels of methylmercury can inhibit neuronal differentiation of neural stem cells."[130] Depression has recently been associated with long-term mercury exposure in former mercury miners[131] and workers in a florescent lamp factory.[132] Additionally, exposure to both arsenic[133] and manganese[134] has been linked to depression, among other conditions.

A large body of evidence has accumulated on the role of organophosphorus and carbamic pesticides on hormonal function. Epidemiological studies conclude that acute and chronic pesticide exposure is associated with affective disorders, and a causal association has been shown between pesticide use and suicide.[135-137]

The harmful effects of substances produced by fungi, especially molds, are now being elucidated. Ochratoxin-A is an immunosuppressant mycotoxin produced by species of *Aspergillus* and *Penicillium* in a wide variety of climates and geographical regions. This compound damages the CNS through a complex mechanism that includes evocation of oxidative stress, bioenergetic compromise, inhibition of protein synthesis, production of DNA single-strand breaks, and formation of ochratoxin-A-DNA adducts.[138] Researchers investigating ochratoxin A's effects on the mouse brain recently concluded, "Overall, these results lead to speculation that ochratoxin-A exposure may contribute to impaired hippocampal neurogenesis in vivo, resulting in depression and memory deficits, conditions reported to be linked to mycotoxin exposure in humans."[139]

Oxidative/Reductive Homeodynamics

A chief complaint of depressed patients is low energy. Ultimately, energy production occurs at the level of the mitochondria in various tissues of the body, and we know that oxidative stress can impair mitochondria functioning.[140] In addition, oxidative stress increases inflammation and cytokine production, initiating a cascade that impacts endocrine and CNS function. A recent literature review[141] found a solid foundation for the hypothesis that oxidative mechanisms serve as a unifying pathogenesis in psychiatric disorders, including depression.

Moretti et al reported:

"There is increasing evidence that affective disorders are associated with dysfunction of neurotransmitter postsynaptic transduction pathways and that chronic treatment with clinically active drugs results in adaptive modification of these pathways... Despite some inconsistencies, PET and SPECT studies suggest low activity in cortical (especially frontal) regions in depressed patients, both unipolar and bipolar, and normal or increased activity in the manic pole. Preliminary MRS studies indicate some alterations in brain metabolism, with reduced creatine phosphate and ATP level in the brain of patients with affective disorders."[142]

Other studies have suggested that mitochondrial dysfunction is an important component of bipolar disorder.[143] Energy transduction dysregulation may involve the enzymatic systems of the Krebs cycle, the electron transfer chain, oxidative phosphorylation, or the enzyme activities of ATP-requiring ATPases.

A recent study examined the possibility that oxidative stress might contribute to the PFC and hippocampal volume reductions that have consistently been found in patients with recurrent depressive disorder. The concentration of copper/zinc superoxide dismutase was significantly increased in postmortem PFC, but not hippocampal, tissue in depressed patients vs. controls.[144] Other investigations have found significantly higher plasma malondialdehyde, adenosine deaminase, xanthine oxidase, and susceptibility of red blood cells to oxidation in depressed patients than in controls. Researchers recently reported that red blood cell superoxide dismutase activity was significantly increased in depressed patients and that there was a positive correlation between severity of the disease and superoxide dismutase activity.[145]

Fluoxetine,[146] escitalopram,[147] venlafaxine[148] and other psychiatric drugs have been shown to reverse or prevent oxidative damage in depression-induced rats. Interestingly, fluoxetine and turmeric had similar efficacy in preventing restraint stress-induced oxidative damage in one study.[146] Taken together, the science indicates that reducing oxidative stress and increasing antioxidant defenses can play a role in depression treatment.

Structural Integrity

In general, the literature indicates that people who participate in physical activity are less likely either to have depression or to develop depression in the future. A 2006 review article reported, "We confirm that there is irrefutable evidence of the effectiveness of regular physical activity in the primary and secondary prevention of several chronic diseases (e.g., cardiovascular disease, diabetes, cancer, hypertension, obesity, depression and osteoporosis) and premature death."[149] Unsurprisingly, all of these chronic diseases are connected through the mechanisms described in this discussion, as well as through their comorbidity with depression, as presented in Chapter 3.

A key factor in the preventive quality of exercise is its acute and chronic anti-inflammatory effect. Although the mechanisms for this anti-inflammatory effect have not yet been fully elucidated, several compelling mechanisms presented in another review[150] include loss of body fat, reductions in macrophage accumulation in adipose tissue, altered macrophage phenotype in adipose tissue, exercise-induced muscle production of IL-6, and alterations in the balance between the sympathetic and parasympathetic nervous systems.

In particular, aerobic exercise at a dose consistent with public health recommendations (17.5 kcal per kilogram per week) was found to be an effective treatment for major depressive disorder of mild to moderate severity in a comprehensive RCT.[151] To give a real world example of this exercise dose, a man weighing 70 kg (154 lb) exercising to a heart rate of 145 beats per minute on a treadmill expends approximately 350 kcal in 30 minutes, requiring approximately 100 minutes of exercise per week.[152] In 2 studies on one population, aerobic exercise was as effective as sertraline in treating depression and more effective at preventing relapse.[152-154] Examining the effects of exercise on mental health in general, a more recent study found that relative increases in maximal cardiorespiratory fitness and habitual physical activity were cross-sectionally associated with lower depressive symptomatology and greater emotional well-being.[155]

Research on exercise and depression has concentrated on aerobic training because this type of exercise is focused on elevating the heart rate and expending caloric energy.[156] However, exercise prescriptions commonly include strength training in addition to aerobic exercise. A recent study found that strength training was positively associated with perceived health and modestly negatively associated with depression, anxiety, and suicidal ideation in female college students.[157] The American College of Sports Medicine has also recommended strength training for older adults, noting that it can offset the loss in muscle mass and strength typically associated with normal aging, greatly improving functional capacity and quality of life in this population.[158]

Psychological and Spiritual Equilibrium

We have already described the physiological mechanisms by which stress leads to neuroendocrine-immune changes. Moving further up the chain of events, psychological, psychosocial, and spiritual factors are also crucial elements. Identifying and evaluating each factor affecting a patient's mental health is a great challenge, one that cannot be encompassed in a single monograph. As examples, however, marital stress, job stress, financial stress, personal illness, and a loved one's death or illness can have a major impact on psychological health. It is clear that stress experienced as a child can cause lifelong disruptions in HPA axis functioning,[159] but the literature also shows that maternal stress can affect the fetal brain, thereby influencing the mental health of children before they are born.[160]

Numerous studies have found that neighborhood context and socioeconomic status also play a role in the quality of health, including mental health. Pathways by which these factors can affect health include:

- Involvement of the SRS as a result of cognitive appraisal of potential helplessness or harm (e.g., low job control)
- Direct effect of health behaviors (e.g., diet, exercise, smoking)
- Neighborhood effects (e.g., availability of municipal services, perceptions of neighborhood safety)
- Social support

A 2003 meta-analysis found that individuals with low socioeconomic status had higher odds of being depressed (odds ratio = 1.81, $p < 0.001$), but the odds of a new episode (odds ratio = 1.24, $p = 0.004$) were lower than the odds of persisting depression (odds ratio = 2.06, $p < 0.001$). A dose-response relationship was observed for education and income.[161] A 1998 study of affluent older adults also found that increasing income level was associated with lower levels of depressive symptoms. However, this association was not statistically significant when measures of health conditions, physical disability, and social support were included in the model.[162]

While the conclusion remains controversial, associational data do suggest that patients who report greater spirituality are more likely to report fewer depressive symptoms.[163] A 2004 survey among patients at an urban primary care clinic indicated that the quantity of one's religious practices were less important than the quality.[164] Quantity of prayer and attendance of religious services did not make a difference in depressive symptoms in this population, yet belief in a higher power, having a relationship with a higher power, and belief in prayer showed significant difference between depressed and nondepressed individuals. The authors acknowledged that lack of faith may merely be another symptom characterizing clinical depression, but they also suggested that among patients whose life pressures can be severe and depression levels high, "encouraging appropriate involvement in spiritual activity or incorporating religious imagery in a therapeutic regimen may have a benefit."[164]

For more complete reviews of psychological and spiritual effects on mental health, please see Liska[165] and Hedaya[166] in the *Textbook of Functional Medicine*.

Nutritional Status

B Vitamins

Many studies show an elevated incidence of folate deficiency in depressed patients; often about one third of depressed patients were deficient.[167] In addition, therapeutic outcomes are worse and relapse rates are higher in folate-deficient patients (see Abou-Saleh and Coppen[168] for a review).

A 2004 meta-analysis concluded that folate may have a potential role as a supplement to other treatments for depression,[169] though it is currently unclear whether that is the case for both people with normal folate levels and those with deficiency. (See *Strategies for Enhancing Antidepressant Effectiveness* in Chapter 4.) A more recent editorial[168] has suggested that 2 mg of folic acid should be given during the acute, continuation, and maintenance treatment of depression. Two articles serving as evidence for this conclusion are:

- 109 patients with major depressive disorder completed a 10-week trial of either 20 mg of fluoxetine with 500 μg folic acid or fluoxetine with a placebo capsule. Ninety-four percent of the women showed a therapeutic response on the folic acid arm (>50% reduction in Hamilton Rating Scale score) as compared with 61% of the women who received fluoxetine only. Men showed no clinical response, but their plasma folate levels increased by less than half of that of the women.[170] Abou-Saleh and Coppen suggested that the 500 μg dose may have been too low to produce a difference in men.
- In a 1990 study, 41 patients with methylfolate deficiency and acute psychiatric disorders received either 15 mg of methylfolate or placebo in addition to standard treatment. The patients receiving methylfolate showed a significant improvement after 3 and 6 months.[171]

Low vitamin B12 status has also been found in studies of depressed patients. In a 2000 study of 700 disabled, nondemented, community-dwelling women over age 65, B12 deficiency was associated with a 2-fold increase in the risk for severe depression. B12 deficiency was present in 17% of women with mild depression (n=100) and 27% of those with severe depression (n=122). A more recent study found significantly lower levels of B12 (and folate) in 33 subjects with depression vs. 33 healthy controls in an elderly community. Homocysteine was also significantly higher in the depressed individuals.[172]

Evidence of B12's effectiveness in treating depression is scarce, but a 2007 double-blind, placebo-controlled study found that supplementation improving B12 (and folate) status reduced depressive symptoms in hospitalized, acutely ill older patients.[173] In addition, another study found a significant association between B12 status and 6-month treatment outcomes for major depressive disorder.[174]

While a complete discussion of mechanisms is beyond the scope of this monograph, the following findings are worth noting:

- A plausible explanation for the association of folic acid and depression implicates serotonin. In most of the relevant studies, low folate deficiency was associated with low levels of the serotonin metabolite 5-hydroxyindoleacetic acid in the cerebrospinal fluid,[167] and in one study, supplementation with folate restored these levels to normal.[175] There is also a decrease in serotonin synthesis in patients with MTHFR deficiency, a disorder of folate metabolism.
- Folate and B12 are major determinants of one-carbon metabolism, in which S-adenosylmethionine (SAMe) is formed. SAMe donates methyl groups that are crucial for neurological function. Folate deficiency decreases SAMe in the rat brain. In humans, SAMe is an antidepressant and increases cerebrospinal fluid levels of 5-hydroxyindole acetic acid (5-HIAA), a marker of serotonergic function.[167]
- Increased plasma homocysteine is a functional marker of both folate and B12 deficiency, and increased homocysteine levels are found in depressed patients. Furthermore, the MTHFR C677T polymorphism that impairs homocysteine metabolism is shown to be overrepresented among depressive patients. (See Folstein et al,[176] Frankenburg,[177] and Coppen and Bolander-Gouaille[178] for discussions of the *homocysteine hypothesis of depression*.) According to Folstein et al, "The homocysteine hypothesis for depression, if true, would mandate inclusions of imaging studies for cerebrovascular disease and measures of homocysteine, folate, B12, and B6 in the clinical evaluation of older depressed patients."[176]

Omega-3 Fatty Acids

Evidence suggests that a significant inverse relationship exists between prevalence of major depression and annual consumption of fish,[179] the prime source for 2 key omega-3 polyunsaturated fatty acids, eicosapentaenoic acid (EPA) and docosahexaenoic acid (DHA). Patients with major depressive disorder exhibit lower levels of omega-3 fatty acids than controls, and there are relationships within these populations between severity of depressive symptoms and lower plasma levels of omega-3 fatty acids. In addition, the ratio between omega-6 and omega-3 fatty acids in the diet may influence the proinflammatory response to stressors,[180] and high omega-6–omega-3 ratios may enhance the risk for both depression and inflammatory diseases.[181]

In 2006, Freeman et al[182] participated in a consensus conference on the role of omega-3 fatty acid treatment in psychiatric disorders (the conference was convened under the auspices of the Committee on Research on Psychiatric Treatments of the American Psychiatric Association). After an exhaustive examination of the evidence, the committee concluded that "the preponderance of epidemiological and tissue compositional studies supports a protective effect of omega-3 essential fatty acid intake, particularly eicosapentaenoic acid (EPA) and docosahexaenoic acid (DHA), in mood disorders." Table 6.1 provides clinical recommendations for omega-3 fatty acids from the American Psychiatric Association.

Biological mechanisms[183, 184] that may explain the impact of omega-3 fatty acids in psychiatric disorders include:

- Increased serotonergic neurotransmission
- Alterations in dopaminergic function
- Regulation of CRH
- Inhibition of protein kinase C
- Suppression of phosphatidylinositol-associated second messenger activity
- Modulation of heart rate variability via vagal mechanisms
- Increased dendritic arborization and synapse formation
- Prevention of neuronal apoptosis
- Improved cerebral blood flow
- Regulation of gene expression
- Competition of EPA with arachidonic acid for enzymatic action and resultant reduction of the inflammatory response

Of the four RCTs that have been conducted to date, three have reported significant improvement in the treatment of depression after omega-3 fatty acid supplementation compared with nonsupplemented controls. The successful trials utilized either 98% pure ethyl ester EPA without DHA or a combination of EPA and DHA as an adjunctive treatment for antidepressant-refractory major depressive disorder. Dosages used were 1 g/d to 2 g/d of EPA alone or a higher dose in combination with DHA (9.6 g/d total). Treatment responses were rapid (as little as 2 weeks), effect sizes were large, and no significant adverse side effects were reported.[182, 185, 186]

In studies of the effects of fish oil on other forms of depression, results have been inconsistent for bipolar disorder, and a lack of effect has been found for perinatal disorder. Studies to date have not supported the use of DHA alone or of alpha-linolenic acid as an intervention in psychiatric disorders.[182]

Magnesium

Magnesium affects all elements of the HPA axis—it can suppress hippocampal kindling, reduce the release of ACTH, and affect adrenocortical sensitivity to ACTH. A 2002 review discussed magnesium's involvement in the pathophysiology of depression:

"The role of magnesium in the central nervous system could be mediated via the N-methyl-D-aspartate-antagonistic, gamma-aminobutyric acid-agonistic or angiotensin II-antagonistic property of this ion. A direct impact of magnesium on the function of the transport protein p-glycoprotein at the level of the blood-brain barrier has also been demonstrated, possibly influencing the access of corticosteroids to the brain. Furthermore, magnesium dampens the calciumion-proteinkinase C related neuro-transmission and stimulates the Na-K-ATPase."[187]

Table 6.1—Omega-3 Fatty Acid Subcommittee, Recommendations Committee on Research on Psychiatric Treatments, The American Psychiatric Association[182]

All adults should eat fish $\geq$ 2 times per week.

Patients with mood, impulse-control, or psychotic disorders should consume 1 g EPA + DHA per day.

A supplement may be useful in patients with mood disorders (1–9 g per day). Use of > 3 g per day should be monitored by a physician.

Adapted from the American Heart Association recommendations to provide guidelines on omega-3 fatty acid use in the context of treating psychiatric disorders

Many studies have shown that magnesium deficiency induces depression- and anxiety-like behavior in rats and mice.[188] Furthermore, magnesium reduced the immobility time in a forced swimming test, suggesting antidepressant effects.[189, 190] In a 2005 experiment, magnesium doses ineffective per se given jointly with ineffective doses of imipramine resulted in a potent reduction in immobility time.[191] Involvement of the NMDA/glutamate pathway was suggested by antagonism of magnesium-induced antidepressant-like activity by NMDA, as well as significant reduction of immobility time induced by a combination of ineffective doses of both NMDA antagonists and magnesium.

In humans, significantly lower serum magnesium levels have been found among depressed vs. control diabetic patients.[192] "Magnesium treatment is hypothesized to be effective in treating major depression resulting from intraneuronal magnesium deficits. These magnesium ion neuronal deficits may be induced by stress hormones, excessive dietary calcium as well as dietary deficiencies of magnesium." Rapid recovery (less than 7 days) from major depression using 125 to 300 mg of magnesium (as glycinate and taurinate) with each meal and at bedtime has been shown.[193]

Vitamin D

While the classic function of vitamin D is to regulate calcium homeostasis and thus bone formation and resorption, we now know that Th1 and Th2 cells are direct targets of the active form, 1,25-dihydroxy vitamin D3, which has been shown to inhibit the development of autoimmune diseases such as inflammatory bowel disease.[194] Vitamin D- or vitamin D receptor-deficient rats have elevated Th1 cell-associated cytokine production and decreased Th2 cell IL-4 secretion. In addition, vitamin D has a neuroprotective role in hippocampal cell survival and may mitigate processes related to cellular homeostasis, possibly through a calcium-buffering mechanism.[195] Other biological effects include synthesizing neurotrophic factors and at least one enzyme involved in neurotransmitter synthesis, inhibiting the synthesis of inducible nitric oxide synthase, and increasing glutathione levels, suggesting a role for the hormone in brain detoxification pathways. Low levels of vitamin D have been associated with mood disorders in the elderly.[196]

A 2007 review article by Michael Holick,[197] one of the world's experts on vitamin D, mentions the association between vitamin D deficiency and mood disorders. His treatment recommendation for vitamin D deficiency is "50,000 IU of vitamin D2 every wk for 8 weeks; repeat for another 8 wk if 25-hydroxyvitamin D <30 ng/ml. The goal is to achieve concentrations of 25-hydroxyvitamin D at about 30 to 60 ng per milliliter." Unfortunately, there have been no RCTs of vitamin D as a primary treatment for diagnosed depression; a MESH search linking depression, treatment, and vitamin D on PubMed turned up only 5 citations, and all but 2 were published prior to 2000. Of those two, one was an RCT of women 70 years old or more (not diagnosed with depression), supplemented with 800 IU of vitamin D plus calcium, in which the treatment arm "did not lead to an improvement in mental health scores."[198] The other was a very small study (15 subjects) of short duration (1 month) comparing vitamin D therapy (100,000 IU) with phototherapy for SAD; all subjects receiving vitamin D improved in all outcome measures, while those receiving phototherapy showed no significant improvement.[199] Clearly, the scientific community needs to explore this issue in far greater depth because vitamin D is intricately linked to many other chronic diseases that are also associated with depression (osteoporosis, cardiovascular disease, multiple sclerosis, and others[197]). It seems a reasonable hypothesis that an underlying vitamin D deficiency (or significant insufficiency) may be one of the web-like interconnections contributing to both emotional and physical dysfunction.

Zinc

Zinc is present in particularly large concentrations in the mammalian brain, and several studies have found lower serum zinc levels in subjects suffering from major depression vs. non-depressed controls.[200-203] A 2006 study found lower levels of zinc in postpartum depression.[204] Low levels of zinc are associated with both markers of the inflammatory response (e.g., increased CD4+/CD8+ T cell ratio, serum neopterin, increased serum IL-6) and treatment-resistant depression.[205-207] However, it is also well established that zinc deficiency impairs some aspects of immunity, indicating a more complex role in the mechanism of psychopathology and treatment of depression.[207] Low serum zinc in depression may be secondary to both lower albumin and "sequestration of metallothionein in the liver, which may be related to increased production of IL-6."[208] Animal data strongly suggest antidepressant activity of zinc, and a preliminary placebo-controlled, double-blind pilot study of zinc supplementation in antidepressant therapy showed significantly reduced symptoms in patients with major depression after 6 and 12 weeks.[209] Possible mechanisms[207] for the antidepressant activity of zinc include: (1) direct antagonism of the NMDA receptor,[210] (2) antagonism of group I metabotropic glutamate receptors[211] or potentiation of AMPA receptors,[212] both of which may attenuate the NMDA receptor function, or (3) direct inhibition of glycogen synthase kinase-3β.[213]

Other Nutrients

Chromium — A placebo-controlled, double-blind pilot study found promising antidepressant effects of 600 μg/d of chromium picolinate; 70% of the patients with atypical depression taking the chromium and none of the patients taking placebo met responder criteria.[214] In a more recent double-blind multicenter trial, the same dose of chromium picolinate reduced carbohydrate cravings and regulated appetite in a population of adults with atypical depression, most of whom were overweight or obese.[215] Chromium also improved diabetic rats' performance in forced swimming tests, with involvement of serotonergic pathways and potassium channels.[216]

Iron — Mean ferritin levels were significantly lower in depressed vs. nondepressed students in a 2007 case-control study,[217] but another study looking at 6 parameters of iron metabolism and mild depressive symptoms in an older population did not find a similar association.[218] Infants with iron deficiency anemia test lower in cognitive, motor, social-emotional, and neurophysiological development than comparison group infants. According to a 2006 review,[219] iron therapy does not consistently improve developmental outcome, but randomized trials of infant iron supplementation have shown benefits, indicating that adverse effects can be prevented and/or reversed with iron earlier in development or before deficiency becomes severe or chronic.

Selenium — Selenium status may modify mental function. "Glutathione peroxidase, thioredoxin reductases, and one methionine-sulfoxide-reductase are selenium-dependent enzymes involved in antioxidant defense and intracellular redox reduction and modulation. Selenium depletion in animals is associated with decreased activities of selenium-dependent enzymes and leads to enhanced cell loss in models of neurodegenerative disease."[220] A 2002 article suggested that the improvement in depressed alcoholics after a period of abstinence from alcohol might be in part related to the coinciding normalization of selenium status.[221] In an earlier article, the same author observed that selenium is required for appropriate thyroid hormone synthesis, activation, and metabolism and that selenium deficiency decreases immunocompetence and promotes viral infections, possibly providing a link between depression, hypothyroidism, and increased susceptibility to viral infection.[222]

Iodine — The offspring of iodine-deficient rats had significantly reduced blood supply to the dorsal hippocampus and cerebellar cortex, as well as loss of the ability to learn, in 2 recent studies.[223, 224] Addition of iodine to the diet of females eliminated these effects. Mild hypothyroidism induced by iodine deficiency led to increased immobility time for rats in a forced swim test.[225]

Tryptophan and 5-hydroxytryptophan — Abnormalities in red blood cell L-tryptophan uptake have been shown in depressed patients,[226] and in a separate study, nonresponders to antidepressant treatment showed lower maximal velocity of L-tryptophan than responders.[227] A 2002 Cochran review[228] concluded that available evidence suggests both tryptophan and 5-hydroxytryptophan are better than placebo at alleviating depression. However, few studies were of sufficient quality to be reliable.

Tyrosine — Tyrosine hydroxylase, the enzyme responsible for catalyzing the conversion of the amino acid L-tyrosine to dihydroxyphenylalanine, may be therapeutically useful in depression. Tyrosine hydroxylase is the rate-limiting enzyme in the biosynthesis of catecholamine neurotransmitters dopamine, norepinephrine, and adrenaline in the neurons. A 2006 study showed improvement in rats' behavioral despair after systemic treatment with tyrosine hydroxylase.[229]

References

1. Gold PW, Chrousos GP. Organization of the stress system and its dysregulation in melancholic and atypical depression: high vs low CRH/NE states. *Mol Psychiatry.* 2002;7:254-275.
2. Packard MG, Cahill L, McGaugh JL. Amygdala modulation of hippocampal-dependent and caudate nucleus-dependent memory processes. *Proc Natl Acad Sci U S A.* 1994;91:8477-8481.
3. Sterling P, Eyer J. Allostasis: A New Paradigm to Explain Arousal Pathology. In: Fisher S, Eyer J, eds. *Handbook of Life Stress, Cognition and Health.* New York: John Wiley & Sons; 1988:629-649.
4. McEwen BS. Protective and damaging effects of stress mediators. *N Engl J Med.* 1998;338:171-179.
5. Seeman TE, McEwen BS, Rowe JW, Singer BH. Allostatic load as a marker of cumulative biological risk: MacArthur studies of successful aging. *Proc Natl Acad Sci U S A.* 2001;98:4770-4775.
6. Tatum J. Psychosocial influences. In: Jones DS, ed. *Textbook of Functional Medicine.* Gig Harbor, WA: Institute for Functional Medicine; 2005:137-147.
7. Kopp MS, Rethelyi J. Where psychology meets physiology: chronic stress and premature mortality--the Central-Eastern European health paradox. *Brain Res Bull.* 2004;62:351-367.
8. Tsigos C, Chrousos GP. Hypothalamic-pituitary-adrenal axis, neuroendocrine factors and stress. *J Psychosom Res.* 2002;53:865-871.
9. Pervanidou P, Kolaitis G, Charitaki S, et al. The natural history of neuroendocrine changes in pediatric posttraumatic stress disorder (PTSD) after motor vehicle accidents: progressive divergence of noradrenaline and cortisol concentrations over time. *Biol Psychiatry.* 2007;62:1095-1102.
10. Bovenberg SA, van Uum SH, Hermus AR. Dehydroepiandrosterone administration in humans: evidence based? *Neth J Med.* 2005;63:300-304.
11. Wolkowitz OM, Epel ES, Reus VI. Stress hormone-related psychopathology: pathophysiological and treatment implications. *World J Biol Psychiatry.* 2001;2:115-143.
12. Lifschytz T, Segman R, Shalom G, et al. Basic mechanisms of augmentation of antidepressant effects with thyroid hormone. *Curr Drug Targets.* 2006;7:203-210.
13. Fountoulakis KN, Kantartzis S, Siamouli M, et al. Peripheral thyroid dysfunction in depression. *World J Biol Psychiatry.* 2006;7:131-137.
14. Thomsen AF, Kvist TK, Andersen PK, Kessing LV. Increased risk of developing affective disorder in patients with hypothyroidism: a register-based study. *Thyroid.* 2005;15:700-707.
15. Kraus RP, Phoenix E, Edmonds MW, Nicholson IR, Chandarana PC, Tokmakejian S. Exaggerated TSH responses to TRH in depressed patients with "normal" baseline TSH. *J Clin Psychiatry.* 1997;58:266-270.
16. Hickie I, Bennett B, Mitchell P, Wilhelm K, Orlay W. Clinical and subclinical hypothyroidism in patients with chronic and treatment-resistant depression. *Aust N Z J Psychiatry.* 1996;30:246-252.
17. Pedersen CA, Johnson JL, Silva S, et al. Antenatal thyroid correlates of postpartum depression. *Psychoneuroendocrinology.* 2007;32:235-245.
18. Carta MG, Loviselli A, Hardoy MC, et al. The link between thyroid autoimmunity (antithyroid peroxidase autoantibodies) with anxiety and mood disorders in the community: a field of interest for public health in the future. *BMC Psychiatry.* 2004;4:25.
19. Abraham G, Milev R, Stuart Lawson J. T3 augmentation of SSRI resistant depression. *J Affect Disord.* 2006;91:211-215.
20. Iosifescu DV, Nierenberg AA, Mischoulon D, et al. An open study of triiodothyronine augmentation of selective serotonin reuptake inhibitors in treatment-resistant major depressive disorder. *J Clin Psychiatry.* 2005;66:1038-1042.
21. Jackson IM. The thyroid axis and depression. *Thyroid.* 1998;8:951-956.
22. Lojko D, Rybakowski JK. l-thyroxine augmentation of serotonergic antidepressants in female patients with refractory depression. *J Affect Disord.* 2007.
23. Baumgartner A. Thyroxine and the treatment of affective disorders: an overview of the results of basic and clinical research. *Int J Neuropsychopharmacol.* 2000;3:149-165.
24. Srinivasan V, Smits M, Spence W, et al. Melatonin in mood disorders. *World J Biol Psychiatry.* 2006;7:138-151.
25. Pandi-Perumal SR, Srinivasan V, Cardinali DP, Monti MJ. Could agomelatine be the ideal antidepressant? *Expert Rev Neurother.* 2006;6:1595-1608.
26. Goel N, Terman M, Terman JS, Macchi MM, Stewart JW. Controlled trial of bright light and negative air ions for chronic depression. *Psychol Med.* 2005;35:945-955.
27. Eser D, Baghai TC, Moller HJ. Evidence of agomelatine's antidepressant efficacy: the key points. *Int Clin Psychopharmacol.* 2007;22 Suppl 2:S15-19.

28. Amin Z, Canli T, Epperson CN. Effect of estrogen-serotonin interactions on mood and cognition. *Behav Cogn Neurosci Rev.* 2005;4:43-58.

29. Huttner RP, Shepherd JE. Gonadal steroids, selective serotonin reuptake inhibitors, and mood disorders in women. *Med Clin North Am.* 2003;87:1065-1076.

30. Shively CA, Bethea CL. Cognition, mood disorders, and sex hormones. *ILAR J.* 2004;45:189-199.

31. Audesirk T, Cabell L, Kern M, Audesirk G. beta-estradiol influences differentiation of hippocampal neurons in vitro through an estrogen receptor-mediated process. *Neuroscience.* 2003;121:927-934.

32. Zhu BT. Catechol-O-Methyltransferase (COMT)-mediated methylation metabolism of endogenous bioactive catechols and modulation by endobiotics and xenobiotics: importance in pathophysiology and pathogenesis. *Curr Drug Metab.* 2002;3:321-349.

33. Lalmansingh AS, Uht RM. Estradiol regulates corticotropin-releasing hormone gene (crh) expression in a rapid and phasic manner that parallels estrogen receptor-alpha and -beta recruitment to a 3',5'-cyclic adenosine 5'-monophosphate regulatory region of the proximal crh promoter. *Endocrinology.* 2008;149:346-357.

34. Morgan ML, Cook IA, Rapkin AJ, Leuchter AF. Estrogen augmentation of antidepressants in perimenopausal depression: a pilot study. *J Clin Psychiatry.* 2005;66:774-780.

35. Schmidt PJ, Nieman L, Danaceau MA, et al. Estrogen replacement in perimenopause-related depression: a preliminary report. *Am J Obstet Gynecol.* 2000;183:414-420.

36. Soares CN, Almeida OP, Joffe H, Cohen LS. Efficacy of estradiol for the treatment of depressive disorders in perimenopausal women: a double-blind, randomized, placebo-controlled trial. *Arch Gen Psychiatry.* 2001;58:529-534.

37. Smith RN, Studd JW, Zamblera D, Holland EF. A randomised comparison over 8 months of 100 micrograms and 200 micrograms twice weekly doses of transdermal oestradiol in the treatment of severe premenstrual syndrome. *Br J Obstet Gynaecol.* 1995;102:475-484.

38. Gregoire AJ, Kumar R, Everitt B, Henderson AF, Studd JW. Transdermal oestrogen for treatment of severe postnatal depression. *Lancet.* 1996;347:930-933.

39. Aloysi A, Van Dyk K, Sano M. Women's cognitive and affective health and neuropsychiatry. *Mt Sinai J Med.* 2006;73:967-975.

40. Almeida OP, Lautenschlager NT, Vasikaran S, Leedman P, Gelavis A, Flicker L. A 20-week randomized controlled trial of estradiol replacement therapy for women aged 70 years and older: effect on mood, cognition and quality of life. *Neurobiol Aging.* 2006;27:141-149.

41. Goldstein KM, Harpole LH, Stechuchak KM, et al. Hormone therapy does not affect depression severity in older women. *Am J Geriatr Psychiatry.* 2005;13:616-623.

42. Heinrich AB, Wolf OT. Investigating the effects of estradiol or estradiol/progesterone treatment on mood, depressive symptoms, menopausal symptoms and subjective sleep quality in older healthy hysterectomized women: a questionnaire study. *Neuropsychobiology.* 2005;52:17-23.

43. Shores MM, Moceri VM, Sloan KL, Matsumoto AM, Kivlahan DR. Low testosterone levels predict incident depressive illness in older men: effects of age and medical morbidity. *J Clin Psychiatry.* 2005;66:7-14.

44. Shores MM, Sloan KL, Matsumoto AM, Moceri VM, Felker B, Kivlahan DR. Increased incidence of diagnosed depressive illness in hypogonadal older men. *Arch Gen Psychiatry.* 2004;61:162-167.

45. Pope HG, Jr., Cohane GH, Kanayama G, Siegel AJ, Hudson JI. Testosterone gel supplementation for men with refractory depression: a randomized, placebo-controlled trial. *Am J Psychiatry.* 2003;160:105-111.

46. Rabkin JG, Wagner GJ, McElhiney MC, Rabkin R, Lin SH. Testosterone versus fluoxetine for depression and fatigue in HIV/AIDS: a placebo-controlled trial. *J Clin Psychopharmacol.* 2004;24:379-385.

47. Rabkin JG, Wagner GJ, Rabkin R. A double-blind, placebo-controlled trial of testosterone therapy for HIV-positive men with hypogonadal symptoms. *Arch Gen Psychiatry.* 2000;57:141-147; discussion 155-146.

48. Seidman SN, Spatz E, Rizzo C, Roose SP. Testosterone replacement therapy for hypogonadal men with major depressive disorder: a randomized, placebo-controlled clinical trial. *J Clin Psychiatry.* 2001;62:406-412.

49. Wang C, Alexander G, Berman N, et al. Testosterone replacement therapy improves mood in hypogonadal men--a clinical research center study. *J Clin Endocrinol Metab.* 1996;81:3578-3583.

50. Wang C, Cunningham G, Dobs A, et al. Long-term testosterone gel (AndroGel) treatment maintains beneficial effects on sexual function and mood, lean and fat mass, and bone mineral density in hypogonadal men. *J Clin Endocrinol Metab.* 2004;89:2085-2098.

51. Rubinow DR, Schmidt PJ. Androgens, brain, and behavior. *Am J Psychiatry.* 1996;153:974-984.

52. Gurnell EM, Hunt PJ, Curran SE, et al. A randomised, controlled trial of long-term DHEA replacement in Primary Adrenal Insufficiency. *J Clin Endocrinol Metab.* 2007.

53. Johannsson G, Burman P, Wiren L, et al. Low dose dehydroepiandrosterone affects behavior in hypopituitary androgen-deficient women: a placebo-controlled trial. *J Clin Endocrinol Metab.* 2002;87:2046-2052.

54. Grimley Evans J, Malouf R, Huppert F, van Niekerk JK. Dehydroepiandrosterone (DHEA) supplementation for cognitive function in healthy elderly people. *Cochrane Database Syst Rev.* 2006:CD006221.

55. Winokur A, Maislin G, Phillips JL, Amsterdam JD. Insulin resistance after oral glucose tolerance testing in patients with major depression. *Am J Psychiatry.* 1988;145:325-330.

56. Timonen M, Laakso M, Jokelainen J, Rajala U, Meyer-Rochow VB, Keinanen-Kiukaanniemi S. Insulin resistance and depression: cross sectional study. *BMJ.* 2005;330:17-18.

57. Timonen M, Rajala U, Jokelainen J, Keinanen-Kiukaanniemi S, Meyer-Rochow VB, Rasanen P. Depressive symptoms and insulin resistance in young adult males: results from the Northern Finland 1966 birth cohort. *Mol Psychiatry.* 2006;11:929-933.

58. Timonen M, Salmenkaita I, Jokelainen J, et al. Insulin resistance and depressive symptoms in young adult males: findings from Finnish military conscripts. *Psychosom Med.* 2007;69:723-728.

59. Weber B, Schweiger U, Deuschle M, Heuser I. Major depression and impaired glucose tolerance. *Exp Clin Endocrinol Diabetes.* 2000;108:187-190.

60. Lawlor DA, Smith GD, Ebrahim S. Association of insulin resistance with depression: cross sectional findings from the British Women's Heart and Health Study. *BMJ.* 2003;327:1383-1384.

61. Roos C, Lidfeldt J, Agardh CD, et al. Insulin resistance and self-rated symptoms of depression in Swedish women with risk factors for diabetes: the Women's Health in the Lund Area study. *Metabolism.* 2007;56:825-829.

62. Weber-Hamann B, Gilles M, Lederbogen F, Heuser I, Deuschle M. Improved insulin sensitivity in 80 nondiabetic patients with MDD after clinical remission in a double-blind, randomized trial of amitriptyline and paroxetine. *J Clin Psychiatry.* 2006;67:1856-1861.

63. Rasgon NL, Kenna HA. Insulin resistance in depressive disorders and Alzheimer's disease: revisiting the missing link hypothesis. *Neurobiol Aging.* 2005;26 Suppl 1:103-107.

64. Ramasubbu R. Insulin resistance: a metabolic link between depressive disorder and atherosclerotic vascular diseases. *Med Hypotheses.* 2002;59:537-551.
65. Kugaya A, Sanacora G. Beyond monoamines: glutamatergic function in mood disorders. *CNS Spectr.* 2005;10:808-819.
66. Palucha A, Pilc A. The involvement of glutamate in the pathophysiology of depression. *Drug News Perspect.* 2005;18:262-268.
67. Rajkowska G, Miguel-Hidalgo JJ. Gliogenesis and glial pathology in depression. *CNS Neurol Disord Drug Targets.* 2007;6:219-233.
68. Sanacora G, Kendell SF, Levin Y, et al. Preliminary evidence of riluzole efficacy in antidepressant-treated patients with residual depressive symptoms. *Biol Psychiatry.* 2007;61:822-825.
69. Sitges M, Guarneros A, Nekrassov V. Effects of carbamazepine, phenytoin, valproic acid, oxcarbazepine, lamotrigine, topiramate and vinpocetine on the presynaptic Ca(2+) channel-mediated release of [(3)H]glutamate: Comparison with the Na(+) channel-mediated release. *Neuropharmacology.* 2007;53:854-862.
70. Gabriel A. Lamotrigine adjunctive treatment in resistant unipolar depression: an open, descriptive study. *Depress Anxiety.* 2006;23:485-488.
71. Schindler F, Anghelescu IG. Lithium versus lamotrigine augmentation in treatment resistant unipolar depression: a randomized, open-label study. *Int Clin Psychopharmacol.* 2007;22:179-182.
72. Pittenger C, Sanacora G, Krystal JH. The NMDA receptor as a therapeutic target in major depressive disorder. *CNS Neurol Disord Drug Targets.* 2007;6:101-115.
73. Muller N, Schwarz MJ. The immune-mediated alteration of serotonin and glutamate: towards an integrated view of depression. *Mol Psychiatry.* 2007.
74. Witkin JM, Marek GJ, Johnson BG, Schoepp DD. Metabotropic glutamate receptors in the control of mood disorders. *CNS Neurol Disord Drug Targets.* 2007;6:87-100.
75. Haydon PG, Carmignoto G. Astrocyte control of synaptic transmission and neurovascular coupling. *Physiol Rev.* 2006;86:1009-1031.
76. Gold SM, Irwin MR. Depression and immunity: inflammation and depressive symptoms in multiple sclerosis. *Neurol Clin.* 2006;24:507-519.
77. Salminen S, Bouley C, Boutron-Ruault MC, et al. Functional food science and gastrointestinal physiology and function. *Br J Nutr.* 1998;80 Suppl 1:S147-171.
78. Patten SB, Williams JV. Self-reported allergies and their relationship to several Axis I disorders in a community sample. *Int J Psychiatry Med.* 2007;37:11-22.
79. Andreasson A, Arborelius L, Erlanson-Albertsson C, Lekander M. A putative role for cytokines in the impaired appetite in depression. *Brain Behav Immun.* 2007;21:147-152.
80. Joynt KE, Whellan DJ, O'Connor CM. Depression and cardiovascular disease: mechanisms of interaction. *Biol Psychiatry.* 2003;54:248-261.
81. Leonard BE. Psychopathology of depression. *Drugs Today (Barc).* 2007;43:705-716.
82. Leonard BE. Inflammation, depression and dementia: are they connected? *Neurochem Res.* 2007;32:1749-1756.
83. Schiepers OJ, Wichers MC, Maes M. Cytokines and major depression. *Prog Neuropsychopharmacol Biol Psychiatry.* 2005;29:201-217.
84. Goodwin RD, Eaton WW. Asthma, suicidal ideation, and suicide attempts: findings from the Baltimore epidemiologic catchment area follow-up. *Am J Public Health.* 2005;95:717-722.
85. Guzman A, Tonelli LH, Roberts D, et al. Mood-worsening with high-pollen-counts and seasonality: a preliminary report. *J Affect Disord.* 2007;101:269-274.
86. Postolache TT, Stiller JW, Herrell R, et al. Tree pollen peaks are associated with increased nonviolent suicide in women. *Mol Psychiatry.* 2005;10:232-235.
87. Reichenberg A, Yirmiya R, Schuld A, et al. Cytokine-associated emotional and cognitive disturbances in humans. *Arch Gen Psychiatry.* 2001;58:445-452.
88. Dantzer R, O'Connor JC, Freund GG, Johnson RW, Kelley KW. From inflammation to sickness and depression: when the immune system subjugates the brain. *Nat Rev Neurosci.* 2008;9:46-56.
89. Basterzi AD, Aydemir C, Kisa C, et al. IL-6 levels decrease with SSRI treatment in patients with major depression. *Hum Psychopharmacol.* 2005;20:473-476.
90. Johnson AK, Grippo AJ. Sadness and broken hearts: neurohumoral mechanisms and co-morbidity of ischemic heart disease and psychological depression. *J Physiol Pharmacol.* 2006;57 Suppl 11:5-29.
91. Andrei AM, Fraguas R, Jr., Telles RM, et al. Major depressive disorder and inflammatory markers in elderly patients with heart failure. *Psychosomatics.* 2007;48:319-324.
92. Dawood T, Lambert EA, Barton DA, et al. Specific serotonin reuptake inhibition in major depressive disorder adversely affects novel markers of cardiac risk. *Hypertens Res.* 2007;30:285-293.
93. Kling MA, Alesci S, Csako G, et al. Sustained low-grade pro-inflammatory state in unmedicated, remitted women with major depressive disorder as evidenced by elevated serum levels of the acute phase proteins C-reactive protein and serum amyloid A. *Biol Psychiatry.* 2007;62:309-313.
94. Libby P. The biology of inflammation: A common pathway in cardiovascular diseases, part I. In: Jones DS, ed. *Textbook of Functional Medicine.* Gig Harbor, WA: Institute for Functional Medicine; 2005:203-212.
95. Raikkonen K, Matthews KA, Kuller LH. Depressive symptoms and stressful life events predict metabolic syndrome among middle-aged women: a comparison of World Health Organization, Adult Treatment Panel III, and International Diabetes Foundation definitions. *Diabetes Care.* 2007;30:872-877.
96. Lipton JM, Zhao H, Ichiyama T, Barsh GS, Catania A. Mechanisms of antiinflammatory action of alpha-MSH peptides. In vivo and in vitro evidence. *Ann N Y Acad Sci.* 1999;885:173-182.
97. Wang R, Xu Y, Wu HL, et al. The antidepressant effects of curcumin in the forced swimming test involve 5-HT(1) and 5-HT(2) receptors. *Eur J Pharmacol.* 2008;578:43-50.
98. Xu Y, Ku B, Cui L, et al. Curcumin reverses impaired hippocampal neurogenesis and increases serotonin receptor 1A mRNA and brain-derived neurotrophic factor expression in chronically stressed rats. *Brain Res.* 2007;1162:9-18.
99. Xu Y, Ku B, Tie L, et al. Curcumin reverses the effects of chronic stress on behavior, the HPA axis, BDNF expression and phosphorylation of CREB. *Brain Res.* 2006;1122:56-64.
100. Xu Y, Ku BS, Yao HY, et al. Antidepressant effects of curcumin in the forced swim test and olfactory bulbectomy models of depression in rats. *Pharmacol Biochem Behav.* 2005;82:200-206.
101. Myint AM, Steinbusch HW, Goeghegan L, Luchtman D, Kim YK, Leonard BE. Effect of the COX-2 inhibitor celecoxib on behavioural and immune changes in an olfactory bulbectomised rat model of depression. *Neuroimmunomodulation.* 2007;14:65-71.

102. Kumari B, Kumar A, Dhir A. Protective effect of non-selective and selective COX-2-inhibitors in acute immobilization stress-induced behavioral and biochemical alterations. *Pharmacol Rep.* 2007;59:699-707.

103. Demaude J, Salvador-Cartier C, Fioramonti J, Ferrier L, Bueno L. Phenotypic changes in colonocytes following acute stress or activation of mast cells in mice: implications for delayed epithelial barrier dysfunction. *Gut.* 2006;55:655-661.

104. Santos J, Yang PC, Soderholm JD, Benjamin M, Perdue MH. Role of mast cells in chronic stress induced colonic epithelial barrier dysfunction in the rat. *Gut.* 2001;48:630-636.

105. Soderholm JD, Yang PC, Ceponis P, et al. Chronic stress induces mast cell-dependent bacterial adherence and initiates mucosal inflammation in rat intestine. *Gastroenterology.* 2002;123:1099-1108.

106. Yang PC, Jury J, Soderholm JD, Sherman PM, McKay DM, Perdue MH. Chronic psychological stress in rats induces intestinal sensitization to luminal antigens. *Am J Pathol.* 2006;168:104-114; quiz 363.

107. Varghese AK, Verdu EF, Bercik P, et al. Antidepressants attenuate increased susceptibility to colitis in a murine model of depression. *Gastroenterology.* 2006;130:1743-1753.

108. Velin AK, Ericson AC, Braaf Y, Wallon C, Soderholm JD. Increased antigen and bacterial uptake in follicle associated epithelium induced by chronic psychological stress in rats. *Gut.* 2004;53:494-500.

109. Zareie M, Johnson-Henry K, Jury J, et al. Probiotics prevent bacterial translocation and improve intestinal barrier function in rats following chronic psychological stress. *Gut.* 2006;55:1553-1560.

110. Kapadia CR. Vitamin B12 in health and disease: part I--inherited disorders of function, absorption, and transport. *Gastroenterologist.* 1995;3:329-344.

111. Cater RE, 2nd. The clinical importance of hypochlorhydria (a consequence of chronic Helicobacter infection): its possible etiological role in mineral and amino acid malabsorption, depression, and other syndromes. *Med Hypotheses.* 1992;39:375-383.

112. Hernanz A, Polanco I. Plasma precursor amino acids of central nervous system monoamines in children with coeliac disease. *Gut.* 1991;32:1478-1481.

113. Pynnonen PA, Isometsa ET, Verkasalo MA, et al. Gluten-free diet may alleviate depressive and behavioural symptoms in adolescents with coeliac disease: a prospective follow-up case-series study. *BMC Psychiatry.* 2005;5:14.

114. Booij L, van der Does AJ, Haffmans PM, Spinhoven P, McNally RJ. Acute tryptophan depletion as a model of depressive relapse: behavioural specificity and ethical considerations. *Br J Psychiatry.* 2005;187:148-154.

115. Booij L, Van der Does AJ, Haffmans PM, Riedel WJ. Acute tryptophan depletion in depressed patients treated with a selective serotonin-noradrenalin reuptake inhibitor: augmentation of antidepressant response? *J Affect Disord.* 2005;86:305-311.

116. Miller HL, Delgado PL, Salomon RM, et al. Clinical and biochemical effects of catecholamine depletion on antidepressant-induced remission of depression. *Arch Gen Psychiatry.* 1996;53:117-128.

117. Mulak A, Bonaz B. Irritable bowel syndrome: a model of the brain-gut interactions. *Med Sci Monit.* 2004;10:RA55-62.

118. Garakani A, Win T, Virk S, Gupta S, Kaplan D, Masand PS. Comorbidity of irritable bowel syndrome in psychiatric patients: a review. *Am J Ther.* 2003;10:61-67.

119. Hirata T, Funatsu T, Keto Y, Nakata M, Sasamata M. Pharmacological profile of ramosetron, a novel therapeutic agent for IBS. *Inflammopharmacology.* 2007;15:5-9.

120. Hiemke C, Hartter S. Pharmacokinetics of selective serotonin reuptake inhibitors. *Pharmacol Ther.* 2000;85:11-28.

121. Schatzberg AF, Nemeroff CB. *The American Psychiatric Publishing Textbook of Psychopharmacology.* 2nd ed. Washington, DC: American Psychiatric Publishing; 1998.

122. Richard K, Hume R, Kaptein E, Stanley EL, Visser TJ, Coughtrie MW. Sulfation of thyroid hormone and dopamine during human development: ontogeny of phenol sulfotransferases and arylsulfatase in liver, lung, and brain. *J Clin Endocrinol Metab.* 2001;86:2734-2742.

123. Zhu BT, Conney AH. Functional role of estrogen metabolism in target cells: review and perspectives. *Carcinogenesis.* 1998;19:1-27.

124. Hays B. Female hormones: The dance of the hormones, part I. In: Jones DS, ed. *Textbook of Functional Medicine.* Gig Harbor, WA: Institute for Functional Medicine; 2005:215-234.

125. Roberts MS, Magnusson BM, Burczynski FJ, Weiss M. Enterohepatic circulation: physiological, pharmacokinetic and clinical implications. *Clin Pharmacokinet.* 2002;41:751-790.

126. Needleman HL. The persistent threat of lead: medical and sociological issues. *Curr Probl Pediatr.* 1988;18:697-744.

127. Stokes L, Letz R, Gerr F, et al. Neurotoxicity in young adults 20 years after childhood exposure to lead: the Bunker Hill experience. *Occup Environ Med.* 1998;55:507-516.

128. Dumont MP. Lead, mental health, and social action: a view from the bridge. *Public Health Rep.* 2000;115:505-510.

129. Condray R, Morrow LA, Steinhauer SR, Hodgson M, Kelley M. Mood and behavioral symptoms in individuals with chronic solvent exposure. *Psychiatry Res.* 2000;97:191-206.

130. Johansson C, Castoldi AF, Onishchenko N, Manzo L, Vahter M, Ceccatelli S. Neurobehavioural and molecular changes induced by methylmercury exposure during development. *Neurotox Res.* 2007;11:241-260.

131. Kobal Grum D, Kobal AB, Arneric N, et al. Personality traits in miners with past occupational elemental mercury exposure. *Environ Health Perspect.* 2006;114:290-296.

132. Zachi EC, D FV, Faria MA, Taub A. Neuropsychological dysfunction related to earlier occupational exposure to mercury vapor. *Braz J Med Biol Res.* 2007;40:425-433.

133. Zierold KM, Knobeloch L, Anderson H. Prevalence of chronic diseases in adults exposed to arsenic-contaminated drinking water. *Am J Public Health.* 2004;94:1936-1937.

134. Bouchard M, Mergler D, Baldwin M, Panisset M, Roels HA. Neuropsychiatric symptoms and past manganese exposure in a ferro-alloy plant. *Neurotoxicology.* 2007;28:290-297.

135. Gamlin J, Diaz Romo P, Hesketh T. Exposure of young children working on Mexican tobacco plantations to organophosphorous and carbamic pesticides, indicated by cholinesterase depression. *Child Care Health Dev.* 2007;33:246-248.

136. London L, Flisher AJ, Wesseling C, Mergler D, Kromhout H. Suicide and exposure to organophosphate insecticides: cause or effect? *Am J Ind Med.* 2005;47:308-321.

137. Stallones L, Beseler C. Pesticide poisoning and depressive symptoms among farm residents. *Ann Epidemiol.* 2002;12:389-394.

138. Sava V, Reunova O, Velasquez A, Harbison R, Sanchez-Ramos J. Acute neurotoxic effects of the fungal metabolite ochratoxin-A. *Neurotoxicology.* 2006;27:82-92.

139. Sava V, Velasquez A, Song S, Sanchez-Ramos J. Adult hippocampal neural stem/progenitor cells in vitro are vulnerable to the mycotoxin ochratoxin-A. *Toxicol Sci.* 2007;98:187-197.

140. Murray AJ, Edwards LM, Clarke K. Mitochondria and heart failure. *Curr Opin Clin Nutr Metab Care.* 2007;10:704-711.

141. Ng F, Berk M, Dean O, Bush AI. Oxidative stress in psychiatric disorders: evidence base and therapeutic implications. *Int J Neuropsychopharmacol.* 2008:1-26.

142. Moretti A, Gorini A, Villa RF. Affective disorders, antidepressant drugs and brain metabolism. *Mol Psychiatry.* 2003;8:773-785.

143. Kato T. Mitochondrial dysfunction as the molecular basis of bipolar disorder: therapeutic implications. *CNS Drugs.* 2007;21:1-11.

144. Michel TM, Frangou S, Thiemeyer D, et al. Evidence for oxidative stress in the frontal cortex in patients with recurrent depressive disorder—a postmortem study. *Psychiatry Res.* 2007;151:145-150.

145. Sarandol A, Sarandol E, Eker SS, Erdinc S, Vatansever E, Kirli S. Major depressive disorder is accompanied with oxidative stress: short-term antidepressant treatment does not alter oxidative-antioxidative systems. *Hum Psychopharmacol.* 2007;22:67-73.

146. Zafir A, Banu N. Antioxidant potential of fluoxetine in comparison to Curcuma longa in restraint-stressed rats. *Eur J Pharmacol.* 2007;572:23-31.

147. Eren I, Naziroglu M, Demirdas A. Protective effects of lamotrigine, aripiprazole and escitalopram on depression-induced oxidative stress in rat brain. *Neurochem Res.* 2007;32:1188-1195.

148. Eren I, Naziroglu M, Demirdas A, et al. Venlafaxine modulates depression-induced oxidative stress in brain and medulla of rat. *Neurochem Res.* 2007;32:497-505.

149. Warburton DE, Nicol CW, Bredin SS. Health benefits of physical activity: the evidence. *CMAJ.* 2006;174:801-809.

150. Woods JA, Vieira VJ, Keylock KT. Exercise, inflammation, and innate immunity. *Neurol Clin.* 2006;24:585-599.

151. Dunn AL, Trivedi MH, Kampert JB, Clark CG, Chambliss HO. Exercise treatment for depression: efficacy and dose response. *Am J Prev Med.* 2005;28:1-8.

152. Aerobic exercise effective for mild to moderate depression. http://www.aafp.org/afp/20050501/tips/21.html. Accessed Feb. 6, 2008.

153. Babyak M, Blumenthal JA, Herman S, et al. Exercise treatment for major depression: maintenance of therapeutic benefit at 10 months. *Psychosom Med.* 2000;62:633-638.

154. Blumenthal JA, Babyak MA, Moore KA, et al. Effects of exercise training on older patients with major depression. *Arch Intern Med.* 1999;159:2349-2356.

155. Galper DI, Trivedi MH, Barlow CE, Dunn AL, Kampert JB. Inverse association between physical inactivity and mental health in men and women. *Med Sci Sports Exerc.* 2006;38:173-178.

156. Otto MW, Church TS, Craft LL, Greer TL, Smits JA, Trivedi MH. Exercise for mood and anxiety disorders. *J Clin Psychiatry.* 2007;68:669-676.

157. Adams TB, Moore MT, Dye J. The relationship between physical activity and mental health in a national sample of college females. *Women Health.* 2007;45:69-85.

158. American College of Sports Medicine Position Stand. Exercise and physical activity for older adults. *Med Sci Sports Exerc.* 1998;30:992-1008.

159. Van Voorhees E, Scarpa A. The effects of child maltreatment on the hypothalamic-pituitary-adrenal axis. *Trauma Violence Abuse.* 2004;5:333-352.

160. Weinstock M. The potential influence of maternal stress hormones on development and mental health of the offspring. *Brain Behav Immun.* 2005;19:296-308.

161. Lorant V, Deliege D, Eaton W, Robert A, Philippot P, Ansseau M. Socioeconomic inequalities in depression: a meta-analysis. *Am J Epidemiol.* 2003;157:98-112.

162. West CG, Reed DM, Gildengorin GL. Can money buy happiness? Depressive symptoms in an affluent older population. *J Am Geriatr Soc.* 1998;46:49-57.

163. Daaleman TP, Kaufman JS. Spirituality and depressive symptoms in primary care outpatients. *South Med J.* 2006;99:1340-1344.

164. Doolittle BR, Farrell M. The Association Between Spirituality and Depression in an Urban Clinic. *Prim Care Companion J Clin Psychiatry.* 2004;6:114-118.

165. Liska D. Influence of mind and spirit. In: Jones DS, ed. *Textbook of Functional Medicine.* Gig Harbor, WA: Institute for Functional Medicine; 2005:165-168.

166. Hedaya RJ. Stress, spirituality, poverty, and community--Effects on health. In: Jones DS, ed. *Textbook of Functional Medicine.* Gig Harbor, WA: Insitute for Functional Medicine; 2005:669-685.

167. Young SN. Folate and depression--a neglected problem. *J Psychiatry Neurosci.* 2007;32:80-82.

168. Abou-Saleh MT, Coppen A. Folic acid and the treatment of depression. *J Psychosom Res.* 2006;61:285-287.

169. Taylor MJ, Carney SM, Goodwin GM, Geddes JR. Folate for depressive disorders: systematic review and meta-analysis of randomized controlled trials. *J Psychopharmacol.* 2004;18:251-256.

170. Coppen A, Bailey J. Enhancement of the antidepressant action of fluoxetine by folic acid: a randomised, placebo controlled trial. *J Affect Disord.* 2000;60:121-130.

171. Godfrey PS, Toone BK, Carney MW, et al. Enhancement of recovery from psychiatric illness by methylfolate. *Lancet.* 1990;336:392-395.

172. Dimopoulos N, Piperi C, Salonicioti A, et al. Correlation of folate, vitamin B12 and homocysteine plasma levels with depression in an elderly Greek population. *Clin Biochem.* 2007;40:604-608.

173. Gariballa S, Forster S. Effects of dietary supplements on depressive symptoms in older patients: a randomised double-blind placebo-controlled trial. *Clin Nutr.* 2007;26:545-551.

174. Hintikka J, Tolmunen T, Tanskanen A, Viinamaki H. High vitamin B12 level and good treatment outcome may be associated in major depressive disorder. *BMC Psychiatry.* 2003;3:17.

175. Botez MI, Young SN, Bachevalier J, Gauthier S. Effect of folic acid and vitamin B12 deficiencies on 5-hydroxyindoleacetic acid in human cerebrospinal fluid. *Ann Neurol.* 1982;12:479-484.

176. Folstein M, Liu T, Peter I, et al. The homocysteine hypothesis of depression. *Am J Psychiatry.* 2007;164:861-867.

177. Frankenburg FR. The role of one-carbon metabolism in schizophrenia and depression. *Harv Rev Psychiatry.* 2007;15:146-160.

178. Coppen A, Bolander-Gouaille C. Treatment of depression: time to consider folic acid and vitamin B12. *J Psychopharmacol.* 2005;19:59-65.

179. Hibbeln JR. Fish consumption and major depression. *Lancet.* 1998;351:1213.

180. Maes M, Christophe A, Bosmans E, Lin A, Neels H. In humans, serum polyunsaturated fatty acid levels predict the response of proinflammatory cytokines to psychologic stress. *Biol Psychiatry.* 2000;47:910-920.

181. Kiecolt-Glaser JK, Belury MA, Porter K, Beversdorf DQ, Lemeshow S, Glaser R. Depressive symptoms, omega-6:omega-3 fatty acids, and inflammation in older adults. *Psychosom Med.* 2007;69:217-224.

182. Freeman MP, Hibbeln JR, Wisner KL, et al. Omega-3 fatty acids: evidence basis for treatment and future research in psychiatry. *J Clin Psychiatry.* 2006;67:1954-1967.

183. Parker G, Gibson NA, Brotchie H, Heruc G, Rees AM, Hadzi-Pavlovic D. Omega-3 fatty acids and mood disorders. *Am J Psychiatry.* 2006;163:969-978.

184. Kidd PM. Omega-3 DHA and EPA for cognition, behavior, and mood: clinical findings and structural-functional synergies with cell membrane phospholipids. *Altern Med Rev.* 2007;12:207-227.

185. Nemets B, Stahl Z, Belmaker RH. Addition of omega-3 fatty acid to maintenance medication treatment for recurrent unipolar depressive disorder. *Am J Psychiatry.* 2002;159:477-479.

186. Su KP, Huang SY, Chiu CC, Shen WW. Omega-3 fatty acids in major depressive disorder. A preliminary double-blind, placebo-controlled trial. *Eur Neuropsychopharmacol.* 2003;13:267-271.

187. Murck H. Magnesium and affective disorders. *Nutr Neurosci.* 2002;5:375-389.

188. Singewald N, Sinner C, Hetzenauer A, Sartori SB, Murck H. Magnesium-deficient diet alters depression- and anxiety-related behavior in mice—influence of desipramine and Hypericum perforatum extract. *Neuropharmacology.* 2004;47:1189-1197.

189. Poleszak E, Szewczyk B, Kedzierska E, Wlaz P, Pilc A, Nowak G. Antidepressant- and anxiolytic-like activity of magnesium in mice. *Pharmacol Biochem Behav.* 2004;78:7-12.

190. Poleszak E, Wlaz P, Kedzierska E, et al. Effects of acute and chronic treatment with magnesium in the forced swim test in rats. *Pharmacol Rep.* 2005;57:654-658.

191. Poleszak E, Wlaz P, Szewczyk B, et al. Enhancement of antidepressant-like activity by joint administration of imipramine and magnesium in the forced swim test: Behavioral and pharmacokinetic studies in mice. *Pharmacol Biochem Behav.* 2005;81:524-529.

192. Barragan-Rodriguez L, Rodriguez-Moran M, Guerrero-Romero F. Depressive symptoms and hypomagnesemia in older diabetic subjects. *Arch Med Res.* 2007;38:752-756.

193. Eby GA, Eby KL. Rapid recovery from major depression using magnesium treatment. *Med Hypotheses.* 2006;67:362-370.

194. Cantorna MT, Zhu Y, Froicu M, Wittke A. Vitamin D status, 1,25-dihydroxyvitamin D3, and the immune system. *Am J Clin Nutr.* 2004;80:1717S-1720S.

195. Langub MC, Herman JP, Malluche HH, Koszewski NJ. Evidence of functional vitamin D receptors in rat hippocampus. *Neuroscience.* 2001;104:49-56.

196. Wilkins CH, Sheline YI, Roe CM, Birge SJ, Morris JC. Vitamin D deficiency is associated with low mood and worse cognitive performance in older adults. *Am J Geriatr Psychiatry.* 2006;14:1032-1040.

197. Holick MF. Vitamin D deficiency. *N Engl J Med.* 2007;357:266-281.

198. Dumville JC, Miles JN, Porthouse J, Cockayne S, Saxon L, King C. Can vitamin D supplementation prevent winter-time blues? A randomised trial among older women. *J Nutr Health Aging.* 2006;10:151-153.

199. Gloth FM, 3rd, Alam W, Hollis B. Vitamin D vs broad spectrum phototherapy in the treatment of seasonal affective disorder. *J Nutr Health Aging.* 1999;3:5-7.

200. Maes M, D'Haese PC, Scharpe S, D'Hondt P, Cosyns P, De Broe ME. Hypozincemia in depression. *J Affect Disord.* 1994;31:135-140.

201. Manser WW, Khan MA, Hasan KZ. Trace element studies on Karachi population. Part IV: Blood copper, zinc, magnesium and lead levels in psychiatric patients with depression, mental retardation and seizure disorders. *J Pak Med Assoc.* 1989;39:269-274.

202. McLoughlin IJ, Hodge JS. Zinc in depressive disorder. *Acta Psychiatr Scand.* 1990;82:451-453.

203. Nowak G, Szewczyk B. Mechanisms contributing to antidepressant zinc actions. *Pol J Pharmacol.* 2002;54:587-592.

204. Wojcik J, Dudek D, Schlegel-Zawadzka M, et al. Antepartum/postpartum depressive symptoms and serum zinc and magnesium levels. *Pharmacol Rep.* 2006;58:571-576.

205. Maes M, Bosmans E, De Jongh R, Kenis G, Vandoolaeghe E, Neels H. Increased serum IL-6 and IL-1 receptor antagonist concentrations in major depression and treatment resistant depression. *Cytokine.* 1997;9:853-858.

206. Maes M, Vandoolaeghe E, Neels H, et al. Lower serum zinc in major depression is a sensitive marker of treatment resistance and of the immune/inflammatory response in that illness. *Biol Psychiatry.* 1997;42:349-358.

207. Nowak G, Szewczyk B, Pilc A. Zinc and depression. An update. *Pharmacol Rep.* 2005;57:713-718.

208. Maes M, De Vos N, Demedts P, Wauters A, Neels H. Lower serum zinc in major depression in relation to changes in serum acute phase proteins. *J Affect Disord.* 1999;56:189-194.

209. Nowak G, Siwek M, Dudek D, Zieba A, Pilc A. Effect of zinc supplementation on antidepressant therapy in unipolar depression: a preliminary placebo-controlled study. *Pol J Pharmacol.* 2003;55:1143-1147.

210. Harrison NL, Gibbons SJ. Zn2+: an endogenous modulator of ligand- and voltage-gated ion channels. *Neuropharmacology.* 1994;33:935-952.

211. Zirpel L, Parks TN. Zinc inhibition of group I mGluR-mediated calcium homeostasis in auditory neurons. *J Assoc Res Otolaryngol.* 2001;2:180-187.

212. Rassendren FA, Lory P, Pin JP, Nargeot J. Zinc has opposite effects on NMDA and non-NMDA receptors expressed in Xenopus oocytes. *Neuron.* 1990;4:733-740.

213. Ilouz R, Kaidanovich O, Gurwitz D, Eldar-Finkelman H. Inhibition of glycogen synthase kinase-3beta by bivalent zinc ions: insight into the insulin-mimetic action of zinc. *Biochem Biophys Res Commun.* 2002;295:102-106.

214. Davidson JR, Abraham K, Connor KM, McLeod MN. Effectiveness of chromium in atypical depression: a placebo-controlled trial. *Biol Psychiatry.* 2003;53:261-264.

215. Docherty JP, Sack DA, Roffman M, Finch M, Komorowski JR. A double-blind, placebo-controlled, exploratory trial of chromium picolinate in atypical depression: effect on carbohydrate craving. *J Psychiatr Pract.* 2005;11:302-314.

216. Khanam R, Pillai KK. Effect of chromium picolinate on modified forced swimming test in diabetic rats: involvement of serotonergic pathways and potassium channels. *Basic Clin Pharmacol Toxicol.* 2006;98:155-159.

217. Vahdat Shariatpanaahi M, Vahdat Shariatpanaahi Z, Moshtaaghi M, Shahbaazi SH, Abadi A. The relationship between depression and serum ferritin level. *Eur J Clin Nutr.* 2007;61:532-535.

218. Baune BT, Eckardstein A, Berger K. Lack of association between iron metabolism and depressive mood in an elderly general population. *Int Psychogeriatr.* 2006;18:437-444.

219. Lozoff B, Georgieff MK. Iron deficiency and brain development. *Semin Pediatr Neurol.* 2006;13:158-165.

220. Schweizer U, Brauer AU, Kohrle J, Nitsch R, Savaskan NE. Selenium and brain function: a poorly recognized liaison. *Brain Res Brain Res Rev.* 2004;45:164-178.

221. Sher L. Role of selenium depletion in the etiopathogenesis of depression in patients with alcoholism [corrected]. *Med Hypotheses.* 2002;59:330-333.

222. Sher L. Role of thyroid hormones in the effects of selenium on mood, behavior, and cognitive function. *Med Hypotheses.* 2001;57:480-483.

223. Gabrichidze GO, Lazrishvili NI, Metreveli DS, Bekaya GL, Mitagvariya NP. Local blood flow in the dorsal hippocampus and cerebellar cortex in the offspring of iodine-deficient rats. *Neurosci Behav Physiol.* 2007;37:495-498.

224. Tsintsadze TG, Gabrichidze GO, Lazrishvili NI, Metreveli DS, Mitagvariia NP. [Altered ability to learn of rat offspring with iodine deficiency]. *Fiziol Zh.* 2006;52:82-88.

225. Kulikov A, Torresani J, Jeanningros R. Experimental hypothyroidism increases immobility in rats in the forced swim paradigm. *Neurosci Lett.* 1997;234:111-114.

226. Jeanningros R, Serres F, Dassa D, Azorin JM, Grignon S. Red blood cell L-tryptophan uptake in depression: kinetic analysis in untreated depressed patients and healthy volunteers. *Psychiatry Res.* 1996;63:151-159.

227. Serres F, Dassa D, Azorin JM, Jeanningros R. Red blood cell L-tryptophan uptake in depression. II. Effect of an antidepressant treatment. *Psychiatry Res.* 1997;66:87-96.

228. Shaw K, Turner J, Del Mar C. Tryptophan and 5-hydroxytryptophan for depression. *Cochrane Database Syst Rev.* 2002:CD003198.

229. Fu AL, Wu SP, Dong ZH, Sun MJ. A novel therapeutic approach to depression via supplement with tyrosine hydroxylase. *Biochem Biophys Res Commun.* 2006;351:140-145.

Section III

Clinical Applications

Having experienced both the successes and failures of psychiatric treatments since the late 1970s, it has gradually become clear to me[i] that our reliance (since the 1950s) on medication and psychotherapy as the sole options for treatment of depression is inadequate for a large percentage of patients. At first, when I began my work in psychiatry, I was regularly astounded at the rapid and wonderful response of depressed patients to medication and cognitive-behavioral therapy. It was extremely gratifying. I obtained certification in psychopharmacology, and soon, with the advent of the selective serotonin reuptake inhibitors (SSRIs), I became expert at manipulating medications to get maximal efficacy. Often, I would usher a patient through a series of medication trials until we seemed to hit the magic formula. Over time, however, I noticed that multiple medications were needed in more patients than before. The "easy" patients of my earlier years seemed to have vanished; today, for several reasons, most psychiatrists have migrated toward a polypharmaceutical approach for partial or nonresponders—a group that comprises about 50% of depressed patients. (See Chapter 4, *Drug Treatments for Depression*.) The existence of such a large group of patients with unmet needs demands new thinking and new approaches to treatment.

Fortunately, via experiences with a series of patients and later my own brush with chronic fatigue, I became aware of the functional medicine paradigm. I have used this approach since 1994 and have found that I can often treat patients without medication or with lower doses of medication, reduce polypharmacy and side effects, and usually avoid multiple medication trials. Patients will respond more favorably both mentally and physically if clinicians take the time to explore the vast array of underlying dysfunctions that can cause or contribute to mood disorders. For the past 5 years, an insurance company has been sending me reports comparing my practice parameters with those of my peers. Using the advanced paradigm presented in this monograph, it turns out that I routinely use about half the amount of medication as my peers and have nearly 100% medication compliance. In a retrospective analysis of 23 consecutive treatment-resistant depressive patients referred to my clinic (mean Beck Depression Inventory score of 34), the paradigm presented here was instrumental in reducing the mean BDI to 8 over a period of 10 months. Clearly, given both the state of the science for this approach and my own clinical experience—and considering the large numbers of people ineffectively treated with current conventional methods—it is logical that large, well-designed trials using this model should be performed. Given the many associations between depression and other chronic illnesses, the harmful impact of which is evident in unprecedented costs and in human suffering, the potential benefits

---

[i] First-person singular usage in the text identifies the monograph's lead author.

of this new treatment model may well extend not just to patients with depressive disorders, but to all sufferers from chronic disease.

What follows in these last 2 chapters is an approximation of my own clinical practice approach, using the functional medicine paradigm. It is not meant to be exhaustive, nor do I imagine that it is without error. It is presented to give the reader an outline, a starting point, and an understanding of how the basic science and the many complex influences a single patient may experience are integrated into clinical practice when treating depression. The scientific foundation of this approach has been described in the preceding chapters, providing a great deal of evidence and logical thinking to guide us. However, we also look forward to a time when studies on complex, individualized functional medicine treatments are funded and reported widely.

Chapter 7

Clinical Discussion: Experiences in Assessment and Treatment

In the majority of individuals, depression is the result of a confluence of multiple predisposing antecedent factors (e.g., genetics, developmental influences and learning, environmental exposures, cultural conditioning, trauma, lifestyle) and more immediate triggers (e.g., divorce, job loss, death of a loved one). There may also be mediating factors that make recovery difficult, such as poverty, chronic pain, or other illness. The depressive process is mediated on the metabolic level by multiple chemical messengers including (but not limited to) neurotransmitters, receptors, second messengers, cytokines, neuropeptides, and hormones.

In most instances, the depressive disorder is not precipitated by a single trigger. Rather, it occurs when antecedents (e.g., genetic vulnerabilities) and life event triggers intersect and interact with dysregulated systems and processes. As an individual experiences more episodes of depression, a kindling process is thought to occur[1] in a significant number of people. The ability to be sensitized or kindled is a property of the central and peripheral nervous system in which, over time and repeated exposure, less and less of a stimulus is needed to evoke a given response. Ultimately, as a result of neuromodulation, a response such as depression may occur in the absence of any stimulus.[2] However, this kindling process may be context dependent[3] and thus modifiable by significant changes in one's context.

> **Clinical Pearl:**
>
> The person with depression is in a complex homeostatic state, albeit a disturbed, negative, painful one. The task of the clinician is to develop an understanding of the homeostatic processes (social, environmental, biological) involved and identify the points that require intervention. The clinician must then intervene at *as many of these points as possible at the same time* to re-establish a new, more functional equilibrium. The ability of the clinician to intervene at multiple points often depends on the resources available both to the patient (e.g., emotional, practical, and financial support) and the clinician (e.g., time, staff support). Assessing resource availability, therefore, is critical—the skills for doing this effectively develop over time, as does the clinician's awareness about the impact of sociocultural factors on both the cause and cure of depression.

The Functional Medicine Matrix Model (see Figure 6.1 in Chapter 6) shows how symptoms, antecedents, triggers, and mediators of disease can be integrated in an organized process that simultaneously evaluates underlying dysfunctions and identifies the most disordered systems. This process and the clinical strategies that flow out of it work extremely well for the evaluation and treatment of depression (and many other chronic diseases). The discussions that follow are thus organized using the functional medicine paradigm, which is fundamentally a systems approach.

Clinical Pearl:

Neurotransmitters are built using several essential nutrients (e.g., tryptophan, tyrosine, folic acid, B12, magnesium, copper) that must be available in adequate supply. High neurotransmitter demand (due, for example, to physical/emotional stress or use of stimulants or other medications such as H2 receptor blockers, which reduce parietal cell output and therefore decrease the absorption of B12) increases the need for these essential nutrients. If any of them are in short supply, neurotransmitter production and maintenance of a steady state are impaired. In addition, the breakdown, absorption, and recirculation of the neurotransmitters are nutrient-dependent processes, requiring folic acid and methionine, for example. They are also dependent on enzymes known to be affected by genetic SNPs (e.g., COMT, MTHFR). *Key tasks for the clinician are: (1) to assess the adequacy of diet (nutritional value of the food sources), digestion, and absorption of the key ingredients used to make and utilize neurotransmitters, and (2) to maximize the efficiency with which these systems work, even in the face of genetic limitations.*

Structuring the Clinical Management of Depression: A Systems Approach

The prevailing conventional paradigm for assessing and treating depression focuses exclusively on dysregulation in (a) neurophysiology, as it affects mood, reward, vegetative function, the stress response system, and cognitive function, and (b) psychosocial function. This model acknowledges in theory the possible relevance of many elements of the Functional Medicine Matrix but has not integrated them into clinical practice, despite the large and growing evidence base that would support such a step. In my opinion, there are many reasons for this failure of mainstream medicine to adopt and adapt, including:

- The continuing power of the excitement generated in the 1950s by the impressive results of psychopharmacology, bolstered by the huge profits generated by sales of these medications
- The influence of the pharmaceutical industry on the direction of research into mood disorders and also on medical education, where a great deal of money is in play to advance the pharmaceutical model
- The managed-care model, which has concluded that the use of pharmaceuticals is the most cost-effective treatment for depression (despite the evidence presented in this monograph indicating that more than 50% of people treated with this model fail to recover fully)
- The pervasive sense of time pressure in both individuals and corporations within Western culture, creating demand for both fast food and fast cures
- The success of the acute-care model, leading to inappropriate approaches for chronic illness
- The fact that conventional medicine has long operated primarily from a mechanistic and reductionist model in which all we need to understand human health is to study the individual parts of the human organism; however, a better understanding of health and disease will require of all of us a much more comprehensive knowledge of the interactions and interconnections among all aspects of the mind-body-spirit totality.

As the previous chapters document, there is a substantial body of mainstream research, often ignored by conventional medicine, supporting both the need for and the efficacy of a more comprehensive approach to depression. In this advanced paradigm, depression is conceptualized as *the product of a reverberating, multidirectional dysregulation in various aspects of the Functional Medicine Matrix, encompassing a large number of antecedents, triggers, and mediators.* In a sense, believing and acting as though depression were a serotonin deficiency is analogous to believing that the world is flat. It is only a matter of time before the interconnectedness of our physical, mental, emotional, spiritual, socioeconomic, cultural and ecological systems is reflected in the treatment of depression.

In our new model, a systems approach is used to gather a full picture of the patient's situation. The clinician must circle around the problems, using different lenses with different powers of magnification and focus, different assessment tools, and expanded attention to the patient's story in order to arrive at a fuller understanding of the underlying dysfunctions.

The Interview: Critical Steps in Eliciting the Depressed Patient's Story

First, of course, the basic information must be obtained:

- Current prescribed and over-the-counter medications, including dosages/durations/benefits and side effects
- Supplements
- Vital signs, including height, weight, changes in weight over time, and reported blood pressure
- Full review of systems to elicit any additional and possibly related complaints and conditions

Clinical Pearl:

Frequently, collateral history can be critical in altering the diagnostic impression and prognosis. Many of the interview questions suggested can be very useful in establishing: (1) level of pre-morbid function, (2) level of childhood function, (3) family psychiatric history, and (4) history of hypomania or mania, to be certain one is not overlooking a bipolar disorder. If all the information is not obtainable in person at the interview, it may be possible to speak with someone the patient trusts, preferably someone who has known the patient for some time, to obtain a different perspective and/or additional information about these issues.

Once the basic information has been elicited, the clinician can ask the patient, "If there were one thing I could help you with, what would that be?" Using the answer to this question, the clinician generates a problem list, and then takes the history of each problem. In the case of depression, it is critical to:

- Get a history of the current episode, including a careful assessment of the precipitating stressors.
- Get a clear history of the first episode and discover whether the depression is episodic, with a certain frequency/duration.
- Ascertain the pre-morbid condition (was there low level anxiety or depression already?), and find out whether there was a significant antecedent to the first episode; "When was the last time you felt really well? What happened next?"
- Find out whether there are usually precipitating triggers; the more episodes one has, the less likely they are to be precipitated by events and the more likely they are to be autonomous or kindled.
- Assess all of the symptoms of the current episode, including suicidality.[4]
- Assess whether this is a hyperadrenergic/hypercortisolemic (melancholic) depression or a hypoadrenergic/hypocortisolemic (atypical) depression, or perhaps a combination. (See *Clinical Interventions* below.)
- Discover what treatments have been tried (dosage, duration, response, side effects); having the patient's pharmacy print out a complete record assists in this process.
- Assess the patient's sense of helplessness and hopelessness, and find out what it is centered around (e.g., the need for power/control, the need to be loved or to perceive oneself as loving[5]).
- Assess the level of anxiety and panic, as these are often implicated in suicide risk.

While attending to the above, many other important aspects of the patient's history and condition must also be assessed, as described below.

Temperament

Temperament is essentially inborn and only minimally modifiable by experience and caregivers. It is distinguished from character (self-direction and the ability to cooperate), which is modifiable. Together, temperament and character comprise what we think of as personality. (See *Understanding Biological Psychiatry*[2] for a brief but clinically relevant discussion of temperament.) Certain important characteristics of temperament can be evaluated by inquiring about the following:

- Harm avoidance
    - Does the patient experience increased reactivity to a novel stimulus?
    - Is change difficult?
    - Does the patient avoid change or novel situations?
    - Does the patient consider himself or herself emotionally sensitive or emotionally reactive?
- Novelty seeking
    - Is intense exhilaration experienced in response to a new situation or a novel stimulus?
    - Is the patient a thrill seeker?
    - Is the patient intolerant of structure and monotony, regardless of the consequences?
    - Does the patient like unpredictability?
    - Are the patient's relationships and work disorganized and in flux?
    - Does the patient get bored easily?
- Reward dependence
    - Is the patient dependent on social support?
    - Is the patient a hard, industrious worker who works until exhaustion?
    - Is the patient sensitive to rejection?
    - Does the patient feel that he or she has an "addictive personality"?
    - Does the patient get cravings for things or situations that give pleasure?
    - Does the patient continue to engage in behaviors or relationships that used to be rewarding, even though they are no longer rewarding or are even harmful?
- Impulsivity
    - Has the patient done things impulsively in the past, which he or she looks back on and questions? What are some examples?

Neurotransmitter Function

Different neurotransmitter systems (hundreds of substances are involved in neurotransmission) overlap and interact, so this approach is only an approximation, at best. Table 7.1 provides a brief overview of some clinical correlates of neurotransmitter function. Diagnostic categories, while useful in many ways, are merely labels. A person can have many labels, but perhaps only one or two neurochemical abnormalities. The neurotransmitter assessment should include:

- Serotonin — Serotonin dysregulation is associated with depression, mania, obsessiveness, obsessive-compulsive disorders, trouble changing focus, cognitive inflexibility, anxiety, mood disturbance, irritable bowel syndrome (IBS), migraine, chronic pain, impulsivity, eating disorders, and perfectionism.
- Norepinephrine — Central norepinephrine activity (generated in the locus coeruleus) is increased in melancholic depression, panic disorder, and anxiety; it is decreased in atypical depression and ADD/hyperactivity in a variety of specific areas of the brain (e.g., portions of the prefrontal cortex).
- Epinephrine — This neurotransmitter can be measured in a 24-hour urine test, which reflects total body status; low levels may be associated with low blood pressure, orthostasis, slow pulse, easy fatigue, chronic stress, or inadequate nutrition.

- Dopamine — High urinary (total body) levels are associated with intense anxiety, psychosis, certain cases of obsessive-compulsive disorder; low levels are associated with depressive symptoms (lack of motivation, decreased libido, anhedonia, apathy) and perhaps ADD.
- GABA — Downregulation of GABA is associated with anxiety, panic, seizures, and depression.
- Glutamate — Look for hypersensitivity to MSG, evidence of hyperexcitability, cognitive dysfunction (Alzheimer's, Parkinson's), psychosis, hypoglycemia, seizure, all of which can be associated with excess N-methyl-D-aspartate (NMDA) receptor activation by glutamate.

Table 7.1—Neurotransmitters of Known Importance in Biological Psychiatry

Neurotransmitter	Type	Derived From	Clinical Associations
GABA	Amino acid	Glutamate	The most ubiquitous amino acid in the central nervous system. Involved in sleep, anxiety reduction, muscle relaxation, mood.
L-Tryptophan	Amino acid	Can be obtained in the diet or through supplementation	Promotes sleep, especially when taken with a high-carbohydrate, low-protein meal. Converts into serotonin, melatonin; can be shunted via alternate pathways away from serotonin production. Dangerous when consumed with monoamine oxidase inhibitors or even SSRIs and SNRIs.
Tyramine	Amino acid	Protein	Dangerous when consumed with monoamine oxidase inhibitors.
Glutamate	Amino acid	Protein	The major excitatory amino acid. Excess (e.g., delirium tremens) is associated with neurotoxicity. Dysregulated in psychotic disorders and probably in mood disorders. Linked with nitric oxide function and NMDA receptors.
Dopamine	Biogenic amine	Tyrosine, fats, carbohydrates	Associated with mood disorders, anhedonia (absence of pleasure), apathy, blood pressure regulation, as well as schizophrenia, Parkinson's disease, ADD, substance abuse, tics.
Norepinephrine	Biogenic amine	Dopamine	Associated with blood pressure regulation and necessary for learning and memory. Probably involved in post-traumatic stress disorder, anxiety, and panic.
Serotonin (5-HT)	Biogenic amine	L-tryptophan	Associated with blood pressure and temperature regulation, gastrointestinal function, vascular and platelet function, mood disorders, and a host of conditions mentioned above.

Sleep

The clinician's interview should assess the following:

- Total amount of daily sleep.
- Initial, middle, or terminal insomnia — If initial insomnia, what keeps the patient awake, obsessing, fear, too much energy, pain, hypoglycemia, restless legs?
- Hypersomnia.
- Decreased REM latency — One of the best markers of depression, but also present in narcolepsy; the clinician should ask the patient, "If you fall asleep during a brief nap, might you be dreaming when you wake? Do you remember your dreams?"
- Sleep deprivation.
- Narcolepsy — Extreme daytime sleepiness (e.g., when driving or upset); also may involve sudden REM onset, sleep paralysis (very vivid dreams in which the person is usually terrified and aware that they are awake, but cannot move), loss of muscle control, and family history.

- Sleep apnea — Associated with increased abdominal weight and blood pressure, testosterone use, snoring, waking up with headache, waking in the middle of the night gasping for breath, and central nervous system (CNS) lesions (e.g., vascular lesions); frequently necessary to ask whether bed partners have complained; it is critical to identify sleep apnea, as untreated it can lead to obesity, cardiovascular disease, stroke, dementia, and, of course, low energy.
- Paroxysmal nocturnal myoclonus (periodic leg movements of sleep, PLMS) — The clinician should ask whether the patient has been known to kick at night while asleep, whether the bedsheets are a mess in the morning, and whether the patient wakes refreshed.
- Delayed sleep phase — The timing of the sleep cycle should be assessed.
- REM sleep behavior disorder — Complex behaviors occurring during sleep that can be indicative of central noradrenergic dysfunction and should be evaluated further.

If indicated based on the history obtained through these questions, the patient should undergo the appropriate sleep study (e.g., overnight polysomnography or multiple sleep latency testing).

Family Psychiatric History

- The clinician should make a family tree for both maternal and paternal sides, including as many generations as possible, then question whether each and every family member has had:
  - Moodiness/aggression
  - Depression
  - Physical, emotional, or sexual abuse, particularly in the family of origin
  - Extreme success, perhaps followed by extreme losses (suggestive of bipolar disorder)
  - Psychosis
  - Unusual lifestyles
  - Migraines (associated with depression)
  - Obesity/eating disorders
  - ADD or learning disabilities
  - Alcohol or drug problems
  - Suicide attempts
  - Diseases associated with affective disorders, including heart disease, osteoporosis, or diabetes (see Chapter 3, *Epidemiology and Public Health Impact*)
  - Unusual creativity, which can be associated with mania/hypomania or can be an early sign of fronto-temporal dementia
- The cause of death and age at death for grandparents, parents, children, siblings, aunts, and uncles should be obtained.
- The clinician should ask about the number of marriages and children; frequent marriages can be an indicator of affective instability and perhaps bipolarity.
- The clinician should ask about the patient's home environment as a child. Were the parents in frequent conflict? If so, was it physical or verbal? Who was the target? Was the patient afraid at home as a child?

Personal History

- What was the patient's birth history? Any prematurity, trauma, or colic?
- Were the childhood developmental milestones within normal limits?
- How did the patient do in school?
- Was the patient very shy?

- Did the patient experience separation anxiety to the degree that it was difficult to go to kindergarten, first grade, or summer camp?
- Was the patient able to do homework, or did he or she procrastinate on larger projects?
- Did the patient have many friends?
- Did the patient feel as though he or she fit in with other children?
- Was the patient the target of bullying (social defeat model of depression)?
- How far did the patient go in school?
- What were the patient's hobbies?
- What excites the patient?
- When was the patient happiest in life? What were the ingredients of that happiness (e.g., physical, spiritual, social, intellectual elements)?
- Does the patient have many close friends now?
- What is the patient's social network like at this point?
- What is the patient's spiritual/religious involvement? Is it satisfying?
- Is there a history of physical, sexual, and/or emotional abuse?
- Has the patient experienced frequent or significant moves or social displacement?

Neurological History

Collateral history is extremely important here, and it is absolutely vital to clarify all issues that arise as a result of this portion of the interview. Positive responses to these questions should lead the clinician to wonder about temporal lobe dysfunction, if not an outright seizure disorder (e.g., partial complex seizures without loss of consciousness), and to consider the implications for pharmacological treatment. For example, most antidepressants would cause such a patient to feel agitated and worse, and thus antidepressants would be contraindicated—at least until the temporal lobe dysregulation is stabilized.

- Is there a family history of seizures?
- Does the patient experience rage or irritability in excess or without a clear reason?
- If there is irritability, is it followed by exhaustion and/or lapses in memory?
- Does the patient ever smell things that are not there?
- Does the patient have unusual sensory experiences or spiritual experiences?
- Does the patient feel suspicious of people?
- Has the patient ever have a seizure with a very high temperature as a child?
- Has the patient ever lost consciousness? If so, in what way, for how long, and how often?
- Has there been any head trauma?
- Does the patient ever experience a blank in time? For example, one can ask, "Did you ever have the experience of knowing that one minute it is 2 PM and the next thing you know it is 2:30, and you have absolutely no recollection of the passage of time?"
- Does the patient ever find evidence that he or she has done something but has no recollection of doing it?
- Does the patient ever see or feel things or his or her body (e.g., hands) as being distorted in size so that they appear or feel very large and close up or small and far away?
- Are there déjà vu experiences? With what frequency?
- Are there jamais vu experiences? With what frequency?
- Have there been any MRIs or brain scans? If so, why was it ordered, and was it normal?
- Has the patient ever had an EEG? If so, why was it ordered, and was it normal?

Standardized Depression Assessment

A standardized measure of depression such as the Beck Depression Inventory[ii] should be used. The clinician can get a baseline measure, done by the patient before the initial interview, and follow up periodically to provide an objective assessment of progress.

Conditions to Rule Out

As the interview progresses, the clinician should develop a list of the standard medical conditions he or she wishes to rule out, such as porphyria, tick-borne disease, complex partial seizures without loss of consciousness (temporal lobe epilepsy), sleep apnea, paroxysmal nocturnal myoclonus, hypochlorhydria, pernicious anemia, and small intestine bacterial overgrowth (SIBO), then make a plan for evaluating each condition on the list.

> **Clinical Pearl:**
>
> Be cautious about labeling someone with a personality disorder because many patients successfully treated for their affective disorder do not show any personality disorder once recovered.[6, 7]

Using the Functional Medicine Matrix Model

Collecting, evaluating, and reflecting upon the above fairly standard information should be followed by a comprehensive functional medicine assessment. Through a careful review of the information gleaned from the interview process, patient questionnaires, or other tools (e.g., Beck Depression Inventory), the clinician will begin to identify the systems that are dysregulated in each patient. Table 7.2 provides a list of systems often dysregulated in depression.

Table 7.2—Systems Dysregulated in Depression

- **Current paradigm:**
  - Mood (euphoria/elation vs. irritability/depression)
  - Reward/pleasure vs. inhibition/punishment
  - Vegetative functions (appetite, wakefulness, circadian rhythm)
  - Reproductive functions (libido)
  - Motor functions (impaired coordination/activity level)
  - Cognition (memory, concentration, judgement)
  - Relational characteristics (isolation vs. interaction)
  - Psychosocial characteristics
- **Advanced functional medicine paradigm (systems-oriented perspective):**
  - Immune surveillance
  - Oxidative/reductive homeodynamics
  - Inflammatory process
  - Digestion, absorption, and barrier integrity
  - Detoxification and biotransformation
  - Structural integrity
  - Psychological and spiritual equilibrium
  - Hormone and neurotransmitter regulation

The remainder of this chapter is organized into 3 main topics that will lead to an understanding of a functional medicine assessment:

A — Assessment Strategies
B — Clinical Interventions
C — Practical Implications and Considerations

[ii] The Beck Depression Inventory is copyrighted and can be purchased at harcourtassessment.com; a copy may be reviewed at http://www.ibogaine.desk.nl/graphics/3639b1c_23.pdf.

A — Assessment Strategies

Laboratory and other tests will help the clinician detect important dysfunctions in the depressed patient. Individualized clinical interventions in the areas of the Functional Medicine Matrix (as indicated by the clinical and laboratory evaluation process) will promote improved response and recovery for a significant percentage of nonresponsive and partially responsive depressed patients, when compared with the current conventional model alone.

Comprehensive Workup (Baseline)

The following tests should be done *fasting* in the early morning in all patients with depression.

1. **Blood**
   - Complete blood count (CBC) with differential
   - Chem 24 — Includes liver function (AST, ALT, AlkPhos), electrolytes (K+, Cl-, Co2, Na), glucose, calcium, total protein, calculated globulin, albumin, A:G ratio, total bilirubin, BUN, creatinine, BUN-creatinine ratio
   - Thyroid levels — Free T3, free T4, TSH, and reverse T3
   - Homocysteine
   - Insulin
   - MTHFR genetic polymorphism (C677T polymorphism)
   - COMT genetic polymorphism
   - Plasma amino acid analysis
   - Red blood cell mineral analysis
   - 1,25-hydroxy vitamin D and 25-hydroxy vitamin D
   - Intracellular nutrient analysis for B vitamins
   - Red blood cell essential fatty acid analysis
   - Lipid panel
   - Serum adrenocorticotrophic hormone (ACTH)

2. **Saliva** — Adrenal salivary cortisol index (adrenal stress index, or ASI) measures cortisol and DHEA output from the adrenal glands (measured at 7–8 AM, 11 AM–noon, 3–4 PM, and 11 PM–midnight); test is highly sensitive[8, 9]

3. **Urine** — 24-hour urine test for catecholamines (e.g., epinephrine, norepinephrine, dopamine) and 5-hydroxyindole acetic acid (5-HIAA); the lab should provide the patient with dietary instructions to exclude substances such as caffeine, stimulants, and certain fruits such as bananas

4. **Other**
   - Body mass index and weight
   - 3-day diet history
   - Exercise history
   - Temperature testing — 3 days, 3 times daily (in the first half of the cycle in menstruating females)

Additional Assessment Options (as warranted)

1. **Digestion, Absorption, and Barrier Integrity** (if there appears to be a gastrointestinal or digestive problem)
   - Digestive stool analysis — Includes markers that test for digestion, absorption, inflammation, adiposity, exocrine pancreatic function, dysbiosis, occult blood, ova and parasites, immunology, and pH
   - IgG delayed food sensitivity test

- Dental exam — Has the patient had root canals, which can result in low-grade chronic infections (that the patient will not feel since the nerve root has been destroyed), causing chronically elevated cytokine levels? Does the patient have gum disease or untreated dental caries?
- Breath test[10] — Simple, noninvasive test that can be considered to rule out SIBO, if symptoms (e.g., belching after meals, constipation, bloating, signs of malabsorption, a sense of prolonged fullness after meals) warrant; the breath test measures both hydrogen and methane produced by bacteria in the small intestine, and higher levels of these gases in the breath indicate bacterial overgrowth in the small intestine

2. **Immune Surveillance/Inflammation/Infectious Process** (if there appears to be an immune or inflammatory problem)
   - If infection is suspected, the source/type of infection should be identified (e.g., SIBO, recurrent/chronic sinusitis, tick-borne diseases such as Lyme [chronic Lyme often presents with reduced CD57 cell count], *Babesia*, *Bartonella*, *Anaplasma*, *Mycoplasma*, EBV, HIV, human herpes viruses, hepatitis), and natural killer (NK) cell activity should be tested; antiphosphatidyl serine (IgM) antibodies, MMP-9, angiotensin converting enzyme (ACE), and an elevated 25-hydroxy:1,25-hydroxy vitamin D ratio (see below) can be indirect indicators of chronic inflammation/infection
   - IgG and IgE testing for food and respiratory allergies
   - Erythrocyte sedimentation rate
   - CRP (highly sensitive)
   - 24-hour challenge test for heavy metals
   - ANA or other autoantibodies testing, depending on syndrome, history, and physical
   - Comprehensive digestive stool analysis, depending on history and physical
   - Eosinophil count, platelets (in CBC)
   - Eosinophil protein x and calprotectin (on stool testing)
   - 25-hydroxy:1,25-hydroxy vitamin D ratio — The active form of the vitamin D hormone (1,25-OH) is present in excessive levels relative to the inactive form (25-OH) in patients diagnosed with inflammatory illnesses such as certain autoimmune illnesses, chronic fatigue syndrome, fibromyalgia, and tick-borne diseases (e.g., Lyme disease); evidence suggests that this is due to unregulated production of 1,25-hydroxy vitamin D by macrophages in the course of an excessive Th1 immune response[11]; a ratio greater than 1.5 can indicate an infectious process (e.g., chronic mycobacterial infection, Lyme borreliosis), in which the T helper cell balance (Th1/Th2) has shifted[12]

3. **Detoxification and Biotransformation**
   - Genetic profile of CYP 450 cytochromes — Tests for phase I detoxification polymorphisms to predict and prevent drug-drug and drug-food (or drug-supplement) interactions and to identify those who might not have the expected response to a medication that requires conversion in the body to an active compound; the test will detect both fast and slow metabolizers (e.g., CYP 2D6 and CYP 3A4 polymorphisms)
   - Functional detoxification panel of phase I (CYP 450) and phase II conjugation pathways — Assesses the body's detoxification capacity, using caffeine, acetaminophen, and salicylate, which challenge specific aspects of the detoxification process; these functional assessments also indicate, to a lesser degree of reliability, potential susceptibility to oxidative damage
   - Digestive stool analysis — Assesses enterohepatic circulation via levels of beta-glucuronidase (a deconjugating enzyme produced by pathogenic bacteria)
   - Assessment of exogenous toxins such as mold[13, 14] and/or chemicals related to occupational and other exposures (e.g., chlordane, PCBs[15]) — Tests for chemicals increasingly associated with neuropsychiatric effects
   - 24-hour challenge test for heavy metals — If exposure is suspected[16] based on occupation or the red blood cell mineral analysis

4. **Oxidative/Reductive Homeodynamics**
   - Cellular energy panel — Evaluates organic acids that play a pivotal role in the generation of cellular energy; this test can reveal metabolic distress associated with generalized pain and fatigue, which may arise in response to toxic exposure, nutrient imbalances, digestive dysfunction and other causes; these organic acid metabolites primarily reflect carbohydrate metabolism, mitochondrial function, and oxidation of fatty acids that occurs during cellular respiration
   - Functional detoxification panel (see above)
   - Genetic profile of CYP 450 cytochromes (see above)
   - 24-hour challenge test for heavy metals (see above)

5. **Hormone and Neurotransmitter Regulation**

   a. Reproductive
   - If a problem with male hormones is suspected, tests (at 8–9 AM) should begin with:
     ○ FSH
     ○ LH
     ○ Free testosterone
     ○ DHEA
     ○ DHEA-S
   - If a problem with female hormones is suspected in menstruating woman, tests should include (at 8–9 AM, once during days 3–5 of the menstrual cycle—the follicular phase, and once during days 18–21—the luteal phase):
     ○ FSH
     ○ LH
     ○ Estradiol
     ○ Progesterone
     ○ 17-OH progesterone
     ○ DHEA and DHEA-S
     ○ Free testosterone

   Testing hormones with a salivary female hormone profile will give much more data (about 11 days of data) about progesterone and estrogen ratios[17]
   - If a problem with female hormones is suspected in postmenopausal woman:
     ○ Estradiol
     ○ FSH
     ○ LH
     ○ Progesterone
     ○ DHEA
     ○ DHEA-S
     ○ Free testosterone
     ○ Adrenal saliva test (see above)

   b. Thyroid
   - If baseline thyroid assessment (including physical exam, history, and laboratory tests) is suspicious, further tests should include thyroid peroxidase antibodies, TSH antibodies, and body temperatures
   - If a goiter or nodule is found on physical exam, thyroid ultrasound and referral for possible fine needle aspiration should be considered

   c. Adrenal
- If hypothalamic-pituitary-adrenal (HPA) axis is overactive (cortisol is elevated) based on ASI, signs, and symptoms:
  - 24-hour urinary free cortisol — Rules out Cushing's syndrome (see below if cushingoid appearance) and exogenous steroid use
  - Assessment for pain and hypoglycemia as other causes of hypercortisolism (aside from a hyper-cortisolemic/hypernoradrenergic affective disorder)
- If HPA axis output is significantly underactive based on ASI, signs, and symptoms, ACTH stimulation test at 8 AM to rule out adrenal gland insufficiency (the baseline ACTH done at initial evaluation will probably be elevated)
- If there is a cushingoid appearance on physical exam, refer for further evaluation, which will include:
  - Abdominal CT scan to rule out adrenal or ectopic tumor
  - 24-hour urinary free cortisol test
  - Pituitary MRI should be considered
- If ACTH is subnormal or above normal, pituitary MRI with and without contrast
- If pituitary insufficiency is suggested on any of the other hormonal axes (e.g., panhypopituitarism), pituitary MRI with and without contrast to rule out pituitary microadenoma (present in 2–5% of the population); assess for chronic infection, which can cause a variety of abnormal hypothalamic/pituitary dysfunctions

   d. Glucoregulation
- If a glucoregulation problem is indicated (e.g., elevated fasting glucose, fasting insulin, or indicators of metabolic syndrome):
  - Fasting and 1- and 2-hour postprandial (following a 75 g glucose load) insulin-glucose tolerance test
  - HgA1c if diabetes is suspected
- If there is a problem with sympathetic/parasympathetic balance, heart rate variability test

   e. Melatonin
- For patients with sleep-onset insomnia or sleep phase delay (circadian rhythm disorders), salivary melatonin test

6. **Structural Integrity**
- Sleep study — Can be considered to rule out apnea, PLMS, and decreased REM latency and to assess delta sleep if symptoms warrant
- Exercise type, frequency, and intensity
- If there is a brain injury, EEG brain mapping; neurofeedback and rehabilitation services should be considered
- Sleep conditions (bedding, lighting, noise, temperature, snoring spouse, barking dogs, etc.)
- If chronic pain syndrome, chiropractic evaluation, orthopedic evaluation, physical medicine consultation, and evaluation of job ergonomics should be considered

7. **Psychological and Spiritual Equilibrium**
- Beck Depression Inventory
- Beck Anxiety Inventory
- Yale Brown Obsessive Compulsive Scale
- ADD testing (subjective questionnaire or continuous performance testing such as Test of Variables of Attention, or TOVA)

- Assessment should include:
  - Sources of learned helplessness, social defeat, and trauma
  - Marital satisfaction
  - Job satisfaction
  - Social and job skill deficits
  - Role changes
  - Losses
  - Current stresses
  - Depth psychological issues — Complexes that develop as a result of recurrently experienced trauma, are associated with ineffective stereotypic cognitive-emotional-behavioral repertoires, and are resistant to logical examination and behavior change

B — Clinical Interventions

Types of Depression: HPA Axis Connections

Before we begin our discussion of clinical interventions organized by areas of the Functional Medicine Matrix, there is an overarching issue that has important treatment implications. Two subcategories of depression may exist that are differentiated by the type of dysregulation of the stress response system (SRS), with differences in cortisol and norepinephrine (noradrenaline) output, cortical function, lateralization of pathology, and attendant differences in clinical phenomenology.[18] These 2 subtypes of depressive disorder are *melancholic depression* and so-called *atypical depression* (which, depending on the particular clinical setting, is often more common than the classic melancholic depression). Individual dysregulation may occur anywhere on a spectrum that spans a hypercortisolemic/hypernoradrenergic state (melancholic depression) to a hypocortisolemic/hyponoradrenergic state (atypical depression). In a given individual, there are both state and trait aspects of this dysregulation, and so measures will vary over time, circumstances, and the chronicity of stress. Nevertheless, it is worth understanding the different poles of the spectrum, as it can expand our awareness of both the psychology and the physiology of depression. Table 7.3 shows some of the common characteristics of these 2 types of depression.

Table 7.3—Two DSM-IV Subtypes of Depression

	Atypical Depression	Melancholic Depression
Gender Predominance	F > M	M ≥ F
Age of Onset	Adolescence	Adulthood
Sleep	Increased	Decreased
Appetite/Body Fat	Increased	Decreased
Immunity	Vulnerable to inflammation	Vulnerable to infection
Diurnal Mood/Energy Variations	PM worse	AM worse
Reactivity to Environment	Yes	No
Energy/Locus Ceruleus Activity	Psychomotor retardation, reduced central norepinephrine	Psychomotor agitation, increased central norepinephrine
Heritability	Yes	Yes
HPA Axis Feedback	Excessive negative feedback and HPA axis downregulation	Excessive positive feedback and HPA axis upregulation
Laterality in Prefrontal Cortex	Reduced right prefrontal cortex activity	Reduced left prefrontal cortex activity

Melancholic depression — The classic type of depression is generally episodic, more common in males than females, and characterized by very severe symptoms. This depression is manifested by an intensely sad and hopeless mood and is accompanied by insomnia (particularly in the middle and later parts of the night), weight loss, a diurnal variation in which the depression is most severe in the morning hours, complete loss of pleasure or ability to anticipate pleasure (including sexual), impaired concentration, agitation, and suicidal preoccupation.[19]

This state of melancholic depression has been clearly associated with elevated central levels of norepinephrine and corticotropin-releasing hormone (CRH) and with hypercortisolemia.[20] Importantly, there is a failure to brake the stress response on at least 3 fronts:

- First, the ventral prefrontal cortex (PFC) fails in its function of inhibiting the amygdala and extinguishing conditioned fear responses, as well as to accurately predict whether a given situation will result in pain or pleasure. In fact, both imaging studies and postmortem studies consistently show a decrease in volume of the left subgenual PFC and overactivity of the left amygdala in this type of depression.[21]
- Second, a subset of cells in the paraventricular nucleus (the parvicellular division) appears to become autonomous of negative feedback, releasing a greater arginine vasopressin (AVP)–to–CRH ratio and sending activating signals to the locus ceruleus (LC). With continued stress, the ratio seems to increase. The specific AVP receptors are more responsive to chronic stimulatory input from cortisol, and this keeps the positive feedback loop active. CRH and AVP seem to act synergistically in activating the HPA.[22]
- Third, cortical CRH receptors, which are part of a negative feedback loop at the level of both the PFC and the hippocampal cortex, are reduced in melancholic depression.[21]

Additionally, there is mounting evidence that the release of AVP occurs in the suprachiasmatic nucleus (SCN), which may be associated with seasonal depression and abnormalities of diurnal variation and sleep.[22]

As a result of this sustained positive feedback response, in which the SRS inhibits the PFC and the left PFC fails to inhibit the core SRS, the patient remains in a hypercortisolemic, hypernoradrenergic loop that is often difficult to break unless both the antecedents and mediators of the condition are corrected. Some of the important issues to be addressed in this situation are social and work skills, cultural context, helplessness-inducing situations (e.g., social defeat, reduced response contingent reinforcement), hormonal dysregulation, nutritional deficiencies, and inflammation. Effective antidepressant treatments are known to increase cortical CRH receptors, reduce CRH and AVP levels, activate the PFC, increase hippocampal volume, and reduce cortisol. In some cases, electroconvulsive therapy may be necessary and effective.

Atypical depression — This type of depression has a higher prevalence in women, an earlier age of onset, higher rates of suicidal thoughts and attempts, and associated psychiatric comorbidities (panic disorder, drug dependence, disability, social phobia, childhood neglect, personality disorders, bipolar type II disorder, and sexual abuse). These patients exhibit a reversed diurnal variation in mood and energy, with worsening as the day goes on. Key symptoms that help differentiate the atypical patient from the melancholic are hypersomnia and hyperphagia,[23] possibly due to the loss of CRH inhibition of appetite.[24]

In atypical depression, mood is generally temporarily responsive to environmental stimuli, but the person experiences a sense of inner emptiness that is pervasive. The loss of pleasure (anhedonia) of the atypical depressive is expressed as a difficulty anticipating pleasure (anticipatory anhedonia), but pleasure is experienced in real time (perhaps tied to the dysfunction of the ventromedial PFC, which, when functioning normally, helps one accurately anticipate whether an activity or situation will be rewarding or painful). Rather than experiencing the psychomotor agitation of the melancholic, the person with atypical depression experiences a great deal of fatigue, often referred to as leaden paralysis. Atypical depression is associated with chronic fatigue syndrome and fibromyalgia; however, the 3 conditions are distinct.

Neurophysiologically, it is generally thought that, unlike the melancholic, the atypical depressive exhibits a *lateralized,* centrally mediated (right PFC and amygdala) downregulation of the HPA axis and a central CRH deficiency. According to Gold[25] and the findings of the national comorbidity survey,[23] the genesis of this form of depression may have its origins in relational difficulties such as neglect and abandonment at an early age, consistent with studies by John Bowlby and René Spitz (anaclitic depression) in the 1940s. According to Schore, "a history of cumulative relational trauma (misattunement between mother and infant), or of frank abuse and neglect, represents a growth-inhibiting environment for the maturation of the right brain."[26] The insecurely (abused, neglected) attached infant's stressful experiences with a caregiver who commonly initiates but poorly repairs intense, long-lasting dysregulated states are incorporated into right-brain, long-term, autobiographical memory.[27] The implication here is that the common atypical depressive disorder and its comorbidities, which are rampant in our society, are the result, in part, of the early psychosocial environment of the mother-child interaction, which first causes a right-sided (?PFC) overactivity and actual suppression of the HPA axis and SRS. This lateralization is opposite to that found in melancholic depression.

Treatment implications — Unfortunately, most studies to date have not parsed out these different subpopulations, and there remains some skepticism about the validity of the concept. There is some evidence that atypical depression is less responsive to tricyclics[28] and that melancholic depression is more responsive to them. A consensus has emerged that atypical depression responds better to monoamine oxidase inhibitors (MAOIs, e.g., phenelzine and tranylcypromine).[29, 30] However, with the advent of the SSRIs, the use of MAOIs declined precipitously, as SSRIs were found to be effective in this group of patients. Additionally, MAOIs often require a tyramine-free diet to prevent hypertensive reactions. The newer transdermal selegiline eliminates this problem at the lowest doses. (See *The Third Generation of Antidepressants* in Chapter 4.) It may retain superior efficacy in atypical depression, although this has not been proven.

Psychotherapeutically, based on the differences cited about etiology above, one would suspect that patients with atypical depression are somehow more vulnerable to the quality of the therapeutic relationship (and any misattunements that might develop) and have a greater need for emotional validation, while the melancholic depressives are more likely to benefit from a cognitive-behavioral/structural approach geared to the current situational triggers and rehabilitation. This conforms to the author's clinical experience. However, much more research is needed on these and other important topics. For example, there is scant research on inhibitors of cortisol production (e.g., ketoconazole) and the use of cortisol for melancholic and atypical depression, respectively, although there are some preliminary encouraging results.

Clinical Pearl:

I use a mnemonic to organize my thinking around the Functional Medicine Matrix and to be more confident that I am not missing something important:

PONG DIED

P = psychosocial	**D** = digestion
O = oxidative stress	**I** = immune/infectious and inflammatory
N = nutrition	**E** = endocrine
G = genomics	**D** = detoxification

Although not included in the PONG DIED mnemonic, voluntary physical activity is as effective in mild to moderate depression as medication and results in an increase in brain-derived neurotropic factor (BDNF) in the hippocampus in animals.[31] *Regular exercise must be part of any treatment plan for depression,* unless patients are hypothyroid initially or have some other limitation.

Clinical Management Using the Functional Medicine Matrix

1. **Psychosocial** — As documented in the previous chapters, the best researched psychosocial treatments for mood disorders are cognitive-behavioral therapy (CBT) and interpersonal therapy (IPT). In mild to moderate depression, the cognitive aspect of CBT is the most helpful, while in severe depression, the behavioral aspect is most helpful and the cognitive aspect is of little use (probably due to regional cortical hypometabolism resulting in cognitive inflexibility and impaired executive functions). Compared with CBT, there are fewer studies on IPT, but studies have also found it to be helpful and a good adjunct to other treatments. A newer treatment approach called interpersonal and social rhythms therapy (IPSRT) attempts to regulate daily activities, such as sleep, exercise, and eating patterns, as well as personal relationships, in order to achieve stability; IPSRT has been shown to be effective in management of bipolar disorder.[32]

Clinical Pearl:

Long-term compliance with prescriptive treatments—whether medicinal, dietary, hormonal, or lifestyle—is a well-known problem. Taking a depth psychological approach to these problems can help identify whether psychological complexes (clusters of unconscious feelings and beliefs, detectable indirectly through behavior that is puzzling, illogical, and hard to account for) are preventing logical approaches to compliance problems from being effective. We all have these "complexes," which are behavioral, cognitive, emotional, unconscious perspectives that are usually developed in childhood around some type of repeated trauma or stress. Most individuals are not aware either of their complexes or how their lives may be affected by these patterns. But by uncovering links to these attitudes, patients are often freed to control their own behavior and to partner in their health. For an example, see *Case Study— Tamika* in Chapter 8.

---

2. **Oxidative Stress** — Oxidative stress is frequently associated with immune, inflammatory, detoxification, and lifestyle factors. Once the presence of oxidative stress has been verified, clinicians must help patients address both the causes and the effects. The first step is to identify the sources of oxidative stress in the patient's life, and then develop strategies for reducing or eliminating them. Next, ensuring the presence of sufficient antioxidants will be a key therapeutic strategy. Antioxidant load can be increased by the use of whole organic foods and freshly made vegetable and fruit juices; however, depending upon the degree of stress and the ability of the patient to make dietary changes, it may be necessary to use supplementation (e.g., lipoic acid, zinc, selenium, coenzyme Q10[33]). Reducing intake of simple sugars will also be helpful because there is good evidence that hyperglycemia-generated oxidative stress is at least partially responsible for the development of insulin resistance.[34] Ultimately, chronic and excessive oxidative stress can cause damage to mitochondrial function, resulting in impaired energy in a variety of tissues, including the brain.

3. **Nutrition and Digestion** — Any nutritional deficiencies identified during testing should be remediated through a combination of foods and supplements (unless there are problems with digestion or absorption that also need to be remedied, such as SIBO). In the individual who is vulnerable to depression or nonresponsive to medication, nutrient deficiencies (e.g., vitamins B1, B6, and B12, folate, iodine, zinc, copper, magnesium, iron) can affect normal neurochemical function of the nervous system.[35]

    As discussed in previous chapters, high-dose folic acid (5–50 mg/d), along with adequate vitamin B12 supplementation, can, in and of itself, be a treatment for depression. In addition, folic acid can augment response to medication and—surprisingly—reduce side effects. B12 can be used sublingually (2500–5000 µg), or intramuscular B12 can be used if there is evidence of decreased B12 function (low functional intracellular assay result, higher than the mean MCV with or without anemia). Intramuscular B12 (methylcobalamin

1000 µg/cc, IM) should be given 3 times per week for 1 month, then once per week for 2 months, then the patient should go back to sublingual, unless there is reason to suspect continued absorption problems. Dosage frequency can be adjusted upwards if patients find it useful or downwards if the rare patient finds it overstimulating (in that case, dosage and frequency might have to be reduced). There are reports of high levels of folic acid inducing seizure; while I have never seen this clinically, it is something to be aware of.

Disturbances at the level of digestion and absorption should be assessed and treated using the help of a nutritionist, the 4R program (Remove, Replace, Reinoculate, Repair—discussed in the *Textbook of Functional Medicine*[36]), and other approaches indicated by the full patient assessment.

IBS is often associated with depression,[37] and many patients with depression have a variety of gastrointestinal complaints even if they don't fulfill the criteria for IBS. Assessing delayed food allergies via IgG testing and correction of gastrointestinal imbalances via the 4R program have, in my experience, eliminated more than 90% of these complaints. A secondary but not unimportant benefit is improved immune function and reduced inflammatory burden, both of which are thought to be significant triggers and mediators on a neurochemical level in depressive disorders. Certain methods of hypnosis have been quite helpful in patients with IBS.[38-40]

SIBO is a common condition that is strongly associated with IBS,[41, 42] and it often underlies chronic symptoms of maldigestion and malabsorption, including bloating, gas, constipation/diarrhea, irregularity, and abdominal pain. Without proper detection and treatment, SIBO can gradually lead to nutrient deficiency or insufficiency due to altered gastrointestinal function, which can increase vulnerability to depression.[41]

Clinical Pearl:

A patient who had depression and persistent nutritional deficiencies demonstrated on blood tests and whose blood levels did not correct with diet and supplements was found to have belching, constipation, and bloating after meals. A breath test indicated significant SIBO, which was treated with several cycles of rifaximin, 2 weeks on and 2 weeks off, along with an antifungal and probiotic support. After several months, his breath test, blood tests, energy, and mood normalized. In order to eliminate his constipation, which is often a cause of SIBO, it was critical to address the pancreatic insufficiency demonstrated on his stool test, which revealed markedly reduced pancreatic elastase, a marker of impaired ability of the pancreas to produce digestive enzymes. Following correction of the SIBO, we were able to correct his nutritional deficiencies and eliminate one of his psychotropic medications. This resulted in less sedation and a reduced medication burden, as well as a probable long-term improvement in his overall health.

As individuals age, or if they are on H2 receptor antagonists (e.g., omeprazole), the functioning of the parietal cells in the stomach deteriorates, resulting in reduced production of hydrochloric acid (stomach acid).[43, 44] This has multiple consequences, including impaired digestion of proteins and increased risk of constipation and SIBO. Additionally, reduced absorption of vitamin B12 due to impaired release of intrinsic factor can occur.

4. **Genomics** — A thorough family history will often reveal many relatives with affective disorders or affective disorder-related illness, either psychiatric or medical (e.g., heart disease, diabetes). While a strong family history makes one suspicious of a genetic vulnerability to affective disorder, it does not prove genetic vulnerability because early rearing experiences in these populations are more likely to be abnormal. However, a family history of completed suicide or a violent suicide attempt should alert the clinician to a higher risk of biological vulnerability and suicide, since violent suicide attempts may be correlated with abnormalities

in cerebrospinal fluid 5-HIAA, a marker of serotonergic function.[45, 46] In such cases, a very careful assessment of suicide risk is critical; if suicide ideation is present, one would do well to consider the immediate use of lithium, which is the only medication proven to reduce the risk of suicide.[47, 48] Lithium can be used temporarily to safeguard the patient and augment antidepressant response while the other aspects of the Functional Medicine Matrix are assessed and treated.

Clinical Pearl:

Disturbances in normal gastrointestinal flora, such as overgrowth of yeast, are common in patients with depression, particularly those with atypical depression, because of the tendency to overeat and crave carbohydrates. A recent case of a 28-year-old attorney was striking. She came to me with intense anxiety and panic attacks, as well as a sense of hopelessness and helplessness. A stool test detected the presence of *Strongyloides*, which was treated successfully with ivermectin, 200 µg/kg/d. While the standard treatment recommendation is for 2 days, an extended 7-day course was prescribed by her internist. Additional triggers of her anxious depression involved job difficulties, recurrent illness in her young child, and living in a high-mold environment with her widowed mother-in-law while her home was being built. Each of these factors needed to be addressed. However, there was a quite surprising and dramatic improvement (70%, by the patient's estimate) with treatment of *Strongyloides*, including elimination of her panic (but not her anticipatory anxiety), overall reduced anxiety, elimination of depression, and successful discontinuation of antianxiety and antidepressant medication. Since there was no evidence of disseminated infection, the remarkable improvement was most likely due to hematologic, immune, and nutritional normalization.

In all likelihood, the genetic component of vulnerability to depression is the result of multiple genes of small effect working in tandem with antecedents and triggers (e.g., developmental, environmental, lifestyle, psychosocial, spiritual, cultural influences). A brief review of the functions of these genes does support the central concept advanced in this monograph: *that depression is a disorder which affects and is affected by the entire person and all of the body's major subsystems.* While no single genetic vulnerability fully accounts for the expression of the depressive phenotype and hundreds of gene candidates have been studied, there is statistically significant evidence for 6 susceptibility genes: APOE, DRD4, GNB3, MTHFR, SLC6A3, and SLC6A4.[49]

- Simply stated, APOE is essential for the normal catabolism of triglyceride-rich lipoprotein constituents. APOE has been studied for its role in several biological processes not directly related to lipoprotein transport, including Alzheimer's disease, immunoregulation, and cognition.
- The DRD4 gene is associated with the dopamine receptor. Mutations in this gene have been associated with various behavioral phenotypes, including autonomic nervous system dysfunction, ADD, and the personality trait of novelty seeking, as well as depression.
- The COMT gene codes for the enzyme that helps degrade intrasynaptic catecholamines (e.g., dopamine, catechol-estrogens). Individuals who are homozygous for the COMT Val allele have diminished prefrontal dopaminergic levels and impaired executive function.[50] Adequate amounts of methyl donors such as folic acid (1–5 mg/d) and S-adenosylmethionine (SAMe, typically 200–400 mg, 3 times per day on an empty stomach) can enable these enzymes to function at their optimal levels.
- GNB3 (guanine nucleotide-binding proteins) is a gene that codes for the beta subunit of G proteins. G proteins integrate signals between receptors and effector proteins within the cell. Beta subunits are important regulators of certain signal transduction receptors and effectors. A single nucleotide polymorphism (SNP) in this gene (C825T) is associated with essential hypertension and obesity, as well as depression.

- The C677T MTHFR polymorphism is more common in patients with affective disorders and heart disease.[51, 52] Particularly in those heterozygous for the SNP, impaired neurotransmitter regulation can occur, often manifested in laboratory testing by elevated homocysteine (except in those with heavy metal toxicity). This is easily corrected by use of 5-methyltetrahydrofolate (dosage should be assessed by measurement of fasting homocysteine level) with B12. Such treatments should be instituted on a lifelong basis and consideration should be given to testing other family members.

- SLC6A4 and SLC6A3 code for the reuptake pump or transporter for serotonin and dopamine, respectively. These genetic variants can influence transporter function by various mechanisms, including substrate affinities, transport velocity, transporter expression levels (density), extracellular membrane expression, trafficking and turnover, and neurotransmitter release. It is increasingly apparent that genetic variants of monoamine transporters also contribute to individual differences in behavior and neuropsychiatric disorders.[53]

Clinical Pearl:

Clinically, I have found that patients who are homozygous for the COMT polymorphism often have unusually high degrees of anxiety associated with their depression. Those who are not responsive to folate or SAMe frequently benefit from low-dose neuroleptics (such as quetiapine, 25 mg at bedtime, or even lower) in the antipsychotic category.

Clinical Pearl:

Polymorphisms of CYP 450 systems (e.g., 3A4 and 2D6) can be tested for and should be used to predict and prevent drug interactions and sensitivities. This is particularly relevant today, when many patients are on multiple medications.

---

5. **Immune Surveillance/Inflammation/Infection** — The association of depression with inflammation discussed in earlier chapters of this monograph suggests that the nervous, endocrine, and immune systems are linked as both triggers and mediating pathways. The clinician treating depression needs to learn to detect and assess triggers of the inflammatory immune response via history and physical exam. Triggers can include psychosocial stressors (known to dysregulate immune response), foods, respiratory allergens (e.g., pollen, dust, molds), environmental toxins (e.g., chemicals such as PCBs and chlordane, heavy metals), and infections (e.g., chronic sinus infections, silent root-canal infections, tick-borne diseases).

The treatment will normally include removing as many triggers and mediators of immune dysregulation as possible (e.g., sensitive foods, allergens, infections), improving vitamin D status, recommending the use of appropriate antioxidants, providing adrenal support (e.g., pantothenic acid, vitamin C, zinc, copper, ginseng, *Rhodiola*, meditation, psychosocial intervention), and selecting from among many other potential therapies, such as:

- Food extracts (e.g., *Cordyceps* to improve NK cell activity)
- Anti-inflammatory supplements (e.g., curcumin)
- Anti-inflammatory medications (including physiological, not pharmacological, doses of hydrocortisone, if indicated)
- Antihistamines (though these can worsen depression)

- Antifungals (these can suppress adrenal corticosteroid output, which can be beneficial in melancholic hypercortisolemic depression, but can worsen the atypical hypocortisolemic variety)
- Antibiotics (both natural and pharmaceutical)

A common complaint of people with depression is "brain fog"; treatment of pertinent immune, inflammatory, and infectious factors frequently eliminates this completely, although improving noradrenergic/adrenergic status via supplements such as tyrosine/phenylalanine or stimulant medications can be required. Other inflammatory symptoms such as arthritis, fibromyalgia tender points, fatigue, weight gain, and skin problems may improve, as well.

6. **Endocrine** — These disorders routinely present with symptoms of depression, including disturbances in the autonomic, thyroid, adrenal, reproductive, glucoregulatory, or chronobiological axes. These disturbances may be the primary cause of depression or, more often, the secondary result of a variety of factors, including chronic stress, chronic illness (including cancer), malnourishment, chronic inflammation, toxic burdens, or infectious processes. Whether primary or secondary, these disturbances must be addressed (unless treatment is contraindicated due to the primary diagnosis) in order to help the depressed individual recover full and vital function with as little medication as possible. The general approach can be supportive (e.g., reducing stress; treating inflammation; improving detoxification, digestion, and diet; supplementing with amino acids or minerals), or it can also involve hormone supplementation. The decision about which approach to take will depend on the urgency for recovery and the orientation of both patient and physician. If hormonal supplementation is chosen, appropriate supportive measures should be instituted at the same time.

The various endocrine axes interact on many levels in ways that are not yet fully understood. (See Chapter 6, *Mechanisms and Interconnections within the Functional Medicine Matrix Model*.) With the complexity of these relationships and interactions in mind, let's look now at treating dysfunctions in the individual hormonal axes involved in the affective disorders.

a. Thyroid and adrenal — When treating the patient with hypothyroidism (much more common in affective disorders than hyperthyroidism), one must consider several issues. Adrenal axis function must first be assessed to be certain that cortisol output is sufficient for the patient to tolerate introduction of thyroid hormone, if needed. If thyroid hormone is introduced in the presence of significant hypocortisolism, the patient can experience overactivation (e.g., anxiety and agitation), despite needing thyroid hormone.

If adrenal axis output is abnormal, then the source of the dysfunction must be determined; among the many possible problems to look for are adrenal gland insufficiency, pituitary insufficiency, hypothalamic insufficiency, brain stem or limbic dysregulation, or psychosocial-spiritual dysfunction (e.g., a misattunement in a major relationship).

- If the ASI result indicates reduced cortisol output, the first step is usually to determine that the adrenal gland itself is functioning and responding appropriately; so an ACTH stimulation test should be done. In practice, the results of this test are usually—but not always—normal.
- Moving up the adrenal axis, pituitary function should be assessed. Is the ACTH output normal, low, or high? If it is low, one would wonder about a pituitary microadenoma (present in about 3-5% of the population), particularly in the face of low levels of other pituitary hormones such as FHS and LH; abnormalities in many other hormonal axes could be relevant as well. High ACTH output is suggestive of an adrenal gland malfunction, but can be generated by pituitary or higher center problems and even certain tumors in 12% to 17% of Cushing's syndrome cases. In addition to small cell lung carcinoma, the most common causes of ectopic ACTH production are bronchial carcinoids, thymic tumors, islet cell tumor of the pancreas, medullary thyroid carcinomas, and pheochromocytomas.[54]

- If pituitary function appears normal, then we can move up the ladder of the adrenal axis to consider the role of the hypothalamus. It is worth noting that infection, inflammation, and immune activation (via, for example, chronic mold exposure, chronic sinusitis, and tick-borne diseases) do alter HPA function at the hypothalamic level and should be investigated as part of this process.

- Next, we should consider the limbic (e.g., amygdala, hippocampus) and brain stem (e.g., the LC, a brain stem nucleus involved in panic, and the solitary nucleus, a brain stem nucleus involved in the regulation of anxiety), areas involved in the emotional disorders. The determination of the role of these centers in the genesis of adrenal axis dysfunction is generally based on history. A temporal lobe seizure disorder (e.g., partial complex seizures without loss of consciousness) or post-traumatic stress disorder would involve these pathways and structures and lead to HPA dysregulation over time.

- Finally, an assessment of early life relationships, looking for misattunement (as well as neglect and abuse) between the mother or primary caregiver and the patient will help the clinician to know whether the origin of the hypocortisolism is based in relational misattunement, impaired development of a sense of identity and self, and attendant right hemispheric developmental disorder.[55]

The supportive approach to adrenal dysfunction that is not due to a tumor, a microadenoma, autoimmune disease, or Cushing's or Addison's disease, involves the use of meditation, stress-reduction techniques, elimination of hypoglycemic stress and physical pain, adaptogens (e.g., *Cordyceps*, ashwagandha, ginseng), vitamin C, pantothenic acid, mineral repletion (particularly zinc and/or copper, if deficient), moderate exercise, and encouragement of fun activities, as well as psychotherapy geared toward psychosocial/spiritual issues. Some practitioners use extracts of adrenal tissue with success, although I have been reluctant because of content and quality control issues.

If the supportive measures do not restore adrenal function sufficiently so that thyroid hormone can be tolerated, the use of hydrocortisone in physiological doses of approximately 20 mg/d can be considered. In my experience, many patients with chronic depression that is characterized by frequent relapses and partial remissions in conjunction with demonstrated reduced output of the adrenal axis benefit from use of hydrocortisone. In these patients, energy seems to improve significantly and the increased ability to handle even minor daily stresses is remarkable. (*Safe Uses of Cortisol* by William McK. Jeffries[56] is an excellent reference for those interested in this option.) Patients who elect this option need to be instructed to wear a medical alert bracelet, to take the medicine only as prescribed, and to observe for any signs of excessive hydrocortisone usage such as fluid retention, weight gain, or craving for sweets. Some patients require less than the usual dose, so it is beneficial to start at 10 mg/d. The typical patient would take 10 mg upon waking, 5 mg at 11 AM, and 5 mg at 3 PM, with a fat-containing snack at each dose. In the event of stress, illness, or surgery, the dose should be increased by 25% to 100% for the duration of the stress or illness. The use of hydrocortisone should normally be limited to a period of 6 months to 1 year, at which point the medication is tapered off in a gradual manner following the standard endocrine procedure for corticosteroids.[57] Tapering off hydrocortisone is not problematic, as long as the supportive measures mentioned above are incorporated into the patient's life.

Once the adrenal issues are addressed, the clinician needs to determine whether to use T4, T3, or a combination of the two. This is best determined by looking at the relative levels of free T4 and free T3. It is not uncommon to see patients who have normal, midrange, or high-normal free T4 with low-normal free T3. In these cases, the difficulty is in the conversion of T4 to T3 in the liver (which can be due to several factors), and use of T3 is preferable. In treatment-resistant depression, relatively high doses of T3 can be used, such as 25 µg/d for a week and then 25 µg twice daily thereafter, along with initiation of an antidepressant.[58] Doses this high usually result in high blood levels of free T3 and suppressed TSH, without clinical signs of hyperthyroidism. When one is not working with such large doses, it is best to follow the clinical picture (including temperatures and the relaxation phase of deep tendon reflexes, as well as other signs and symptoms and lab tests) to determine appropriate doses.

Patients must take thyroid hormone in a consistent manner and on an empty stomach away from supplements, all food, and other medications. Adjustment of thyroid doses should always be followed by the standard thyroid panel about 6 weeks later, done in the morning if one wants to determine trough levels of free T3 or about 4–6 hours after T3 supplementation if one wants to determine peak levels of free T3. Excessive doses of thyroid hormone resulting in suppressed TSH may be associated with osteoporosis, and so the cost-benefit balance of such an approach must be considered in each patient. Weight-bearing exercise, regular bone scans, optimal calcium and vitamin D status, reduction of inflammation, and perhaps bisphosphonates and/or vitamin D analogs may help to temper the risk if the patient does need suppressive therapy. Thyroid antibodies also should be tested, including thyroid peroxidase antibodies and, if the patient appears hyperthyroid, TSH antibodies. Patients with Hashimoto's thyroiditis may require closer monitoring and dosage adjustments, as well as supplementation with selenium and attention to adrenal function.

The clinician needs to be aware that a consensus has been developing since the 2002 NHANES study[59] that the standard reference range for TSH is inappropriate. For patients with affective disorders, it is generally best to keep TSH levels between 0.5 and 2.0 mIU/L.[60, 61]

b. Reproductive hormones — Deficiencies in reproductive hormones can arise from several sources, such as nutrition (e.g., low zinc is associated with treatment-resistant depression,[62] inflammatory states,[63] and low testosterone production[64]), stress, toxins (e.g., marijuana reduces testosterone production), pituitary microadenoma, total oophorectomy, or genetic problems (e.g., Klinefelter's syndrome). These disturbances (in both men and women) are clearly associated with depression as both cause (less often) and contributors to treatment resistance. Of course, adrenal deficiency in itself, as well as deficient gonadal output, can be contributory to low reproductive hormones. In males and females, measurement of FSH, LH, zinc, free testosterone (taken as baseline in the morning and on 3 occasions at the same lab to establish low testosterone), DHEA, DHEA-S (preferably via an ASI and blood), and estradiol should be taken.

In older males, PSA and prostate exam are used as part of the baseline measures. If established, replacement of appropriate hormones can be very helpful with mood, cognition, muscle strength, sexual function, and self-esteem. Excessive doses can cause increased hematocrit, sleep apnea, irritability, acne, and male pattern hair growth; therefore, regular monitoring of blood levels of free testosterone (4–6 hours after morning application of gel or patch) is necessary.

The clinician should be alert to certain genetic enzymatic deficiencies in women; for example, 17- and 21-hydroxylase deficiencies are more common in Ashkenazic women of eastern European ancestry. These deficiencies can be associated with reduced cortisol output (and, therefore, intense fatigue, difficulty handling stress, and depression), increased signs of virilization, infertility (polycystic ovaries), metabolic syndrome, and so forth.

Peri- and postmenopausal women with depression have been shown to benefit from use of the estradiol patch,[65-67] but not oral estradiol or synthetic estrogens. Use of the patch can be considered in some patients, taking into consideration the risks and benefits of using exogenous hormones. If used, many gynecologists prefer to add a small dose of progesterone (e.g., 50–100 mg at bedtime) so as to avoid the risks of using unopposed estrogen. The clinician and patient must work with the patient's gynecologist or other primary care provider to assure appropriate medical follow-up.

In the case of depression associated with the menstrual cycle (premenstrual dysphoric disorder or PMDD), the clinician should first document mood and relevant symptoms for 3 months, while collecting hormonal data (as described above) to document the diagnosis. If indicated, based on the data collected, the use of bioidentical progesterone in the luteal phase of the menstrual cycle can be quite helpful, with or without an estrogen patch in place. Again, if using this approach, clinician and patient must work with the patient's primary care provider to assure appropriate medical follow-up.

Generally speaking, it is helpful for the clinician to correct as many adrenal hormones as possible by intervening as high up in the adrenal cascade as possible. Since cholesterol is the mother molecule for all adrenal steroid hormones, many people on statin drugs can develop subtle adrenal insufficiency with reductions in pregnenolone, DHEA/DHEA-S, cortisol, testosterone, and estrogen levels. Cholesterol is converted to pregnenolone, which then is metabolized along multiple pathways in the adrenal gland, and so use of pregnenolone can be quite effective. If used, then repeat testing of downstream hormones (DHEA, testosterone, estradiol) should be performed to ensure that levels of these hormones are within normal limits. There have been both positive and negative studies on the use of high-dose DHEA (e.g., 500 mg/d) in treatment of depression[68-70]; however, use of pharmacological doses of reproductive hormones entails unknown risks. In general, whether one is supplementing with DHEA, testosterone, estrogen, or progesterone, using bioidentical hormones to establish normal physiological levels is the most prudent approach. When testing for DHEA and testosterone levels after supplementation, such testing should be done about 4–6 hours after administration of the hormone. Oral hormones should be taken with a fat-containing snack since the steroid hormones are lipid soluble.

A proper balance between 2-hydroxy estrone and 16-alpha-hydroxy estrone is important for optimal health. Flaxseed and soy products (isoflavones),[71] cruciferous vegetables (indole-3-carbinol[72]), increased lean body mass,[73, 74] and omega-3 fatty acids[75] are interventions that may reduce the risk of estrogen-dependent disease by favorably modifying this ratio. Practitioners should closely monitor the physiological impact of these and other treatments (including the use of the estrogen patch in perimenopausal and postmenopausal women with depression), particularly in those women who are thought to need additional estrogen as part of their antidepressant regimen and who may have risk factors for estrogen-sensitive diseases. A cost-benefit analysis must be made in such cases.

c.   Glucoregulation — Maintaining stable glucose levels appears to be important in management of mood. Treating insulin resistance and type 2 diabetes can show multiple positive results, including improvement in metabolic parameters, the mood disorder, energy, markers of inflammation, and self-esteem. The focus should be on adjusting the patient's diet to (a) eliminate high-glycemic-index foods, (b) provide the appropriate balance of protein, fat, and complex carbohydrates, and (c) moderate caloric intake. Meals should be more heavily loaded (higher caloric content) toward the first two thirds of the day, unless the patient is taking 5–6 small meals per day. In addition, supplementing with plant sterols and appropriate minerals such as chromium (200 µg, up to 3 times per day, depending on red blood cell chromium levels) and R-lipoic acid (200 mg, 3 times per day) and instituting a program of regular, moderate exercise are all very useful interventions. Eliminating any sensitive foods from the patient's diet and correcting any gastrointestinal disorders are also important steps to take. Generally, insulin resistance can be normalized using this approach within 3 to 6 months; it has been effective with over 90% of the patients in my clinic whose conditions warranted this type of intervention. If significant weight loss is expected, it is important that the gastrointestinal and liver detoxification pathways be supported using lipoic acid, milk thistle, and a multi-mineral supplement (or one of a variety of medical food liver/gut support products) because weight loss is accompanied by release of fat-soluble toxins and hormones from adipocytes. Using a behavioral support program to maintain these lifestyle changes is also important. This can involve, for example, periodic follow-up phone calls to the patient, routine check-in appointments, and/or a behavior-modification program with built-in, agreed-upon punishments and rewards.

d.   Melatonin — Given that it is a hormone, melatonin should be used only if low or low-normal levels are detected. Melatonin dosage can range from 0.5 to 10 mg. I suggest measuring with salivary samples, then titrating to a dose that normalizes levels. It is important to recheck and make sure the dose is not too high. Remember that supraphysiological doses of hormones put us in unknown and potentially dangerous territory.

7. **Detoxification** — Hepatic detoxification systems may affect brain function. Therefore, effective treatment of affective disorders must include assessment and treatment (if necessary) of phase I and II detoxification pathways, as well as dysbiosis. Although exhaustive clinical studies have yet to be performed, we have the biochemical and logical basis upon which to recommend interventions in order to help patients with evidence of chemical sensitivity or high exposures to toxic compounds.

It is important to realize that any change in the metabolic clearance of a drug—whether induced by an enzyme, another drug, or a food, herb, or supplement—can result in a change in steady-state concentration that will alter its effect.[76] Knowledge of CYP 450 interactions is essential whether one is treating with whole foods, pharmacology, or herbal supplements. In addition, if dysbiosis is present in the gastrointestinal tract, the conjugation reaction (glucuronidation) performed by the liver is undone by pathogenic bacteria in the intestinal tract, releasing toxins and hormones (e.g., estrogens) which are then available for reabsorption in the bloodstream and CNS, with attendant psychotropic effects.

Liver and gut support can reduce medication side effects, doses of medication, and toxicity and can affect the brain via hormonal and catecholamine pathways, as well as first-pass metabolism in the gut and the liver. Failure to address gut-liver alteration can result in continued dysfunction of hormonal and catecholamine metabolism, treatment resistance, unnecessary side effects, noncompliance, neurotoxicity, increased relapse rates, decreased remission rates, excessive medication doses, and drug-drug interactions.

Clinical Pearl:

Because nutritional modification of the CYP 450 and/or conjugation pathways has strong potential to change drug metabolism, practitioners should use caution and awareness when recommending such strategies in patients taking prescription medications or useful herbal supplements such as St. John's wort. St. John's wort can be recommended when patients express a preference for a natural approach, rather than a pharmaceutical one. Many studies have shown St. John's wort to be as effective in mild to moderate depression as antidepressant drugs.[77-79] However, it's very important to prescribe a supplement whose quality and efficacy you can trust. The Web site www.consumerlab.com can be consulted to check on various products by name.

C — Practical Implications and Considerations

Many clinicians who do not have specialized training in psychology or psychiatry treat depressed patients. It is our hope that this monograph will provide information that can help improve their patient outcomes. However, because depression carries the risk of suicide and has such harmful effects on quality of life, it is critical to be alert to situations in which a referral to a specialist may be indicated for further evaluation or for treatment. I have had experiences in practice that have made me concerned that inadequate training and inadequate time allotted to patient evaluation and follow-up, particularly in the managed care setting, are leading to inappropriate prescribing practices and the inadvertent worsening of depression outcomes, including an increased risk of suicide.

There are several positive potential outcomes of integrating a functional medicine approach into the assessment and treatment of depression:

- Reliance on medication as the primary therapeutic option is no longer necessary; fewer medications may be needed (or even none), and those used will be more efficacious.
- There are many conditions that are comorbid with depression (as discussed extensively in this monograph), and the effects are often multidirectional: depression can worsen the course of other conditions, and other conditions can adversely affect the depressed patient's mood. Acting on multiple major problem areas simultaneously increases the likelihood of improving the depression, improving general well-being, and reducing comorbidities.
- Outcomes may be improved. For example, a study by Coppen[80] with 127 patients showed a significant improvement in response rate (94% vs. 61%, $p < 0.005$) for those on fluoxetine and folate vs. those on fluoxetine alone. Furthermore, the recovery rate increased from 47% (fluoxetine alone) to 73% with the addition of folate ($p < 0.06$). A recent meta-analysis of the association between low folate and depression confirms the finding.[81]
- Side effects may be reduced or avoided entirely. In that same Coppen study, adverse events severe enough to cause withdrawal from the trial and reports of side effects were both significantly lower in the folic acid group ($p < 0.05$).
- A reduced public health burden will result from the lessening of both mental and physical complaints.
- Clinician satisfaction can increase markedly with improved patient outcomes.
- The clinician who pays attention to both the mental and physical health of the patient avoids seeing the patient as *either* a psychological *or* a medical case—a most uncomfortable (and unrealistic) split.

Unfortunately, there are also obstacles to providing this kind of care.

- Most conventional practitioners are educated in an acute-care model, in which the thinking is linear and the goal is to control physiology, rather than a systems-oriented model, in which the goal is to manage multiple interacting factors to improve multiple affected processes.
- Managed care places a significant burden on practitioners, who may have less time for direct patient care and who may also be experiencing financial pressures from reduced reimbursement schedules. Functional medicine requires time—time to elicit the patient's story in depth, time to explore all the elements of dysfunction that are disturbing the patient's well being, and time to restore balance and function. And the short-term cost of both assessment and treatment can be significant if not reimbursed by a third-party payer. The need for studies to document the efficacy of the functional medicine model is urgent; research can drive policy change to support a paradigm shift in both delivery of care and reimbursement.
- Individuals and families, as well as clinicians, are under considerable time pressure. Americans work more hours per year than people in any other developed country, and the economic pressures (perceived and real) that drive this phenomenon are not likely to lessen. Time to exercise (sedentary occupations are now the norm), to eat together as a family, to prepare fresh, healthy, locally grown food, to participate in pleasurable activities, and to make friends and spend time with them is in short supply.
- Depression still carries a stigma. The clinician must engage the patient—via education about biology as well as the learned helplessness and social defeat models—in understanding that help can be provided, but only if all the necessary information for understanding the patient's condition is forthcoming. Despite public education, many patients need reassurance that being depressed is not a character flaw or a moral lapse. It is the result of complex interactions among genetics, biology, experiences, and the environment within which the patient lives.
- Depression itself reduces the inclination for self-care, which is an essential component of functional medicine.

Utilizing the functional medicine approach requires that you listen to the patient, collect a very detailed and comprehensive history, work in partnership with the patient to remove obstacles to self-care, and develop and use your relational/empathic, analytic, and critical thinking skills. There are no algorithms, no one-size-fits-all therapies.

Each person must be evaluated as a unique individual, and the treatment plan must be tailored individually to address his/her particular issues. We have discussed many strategies that will help you meet these goals, but even this lengthy monograph is not exhaustive; each clinician must keep learning and integrating new knowledge on a regular basis to keep the model alive and growing.

Decisions are not made unilaterally in this model; they are discussed between patient and physician. Clinicians should take the time to explain the need for partnership in this approach. Patients are the experts on their own lives, while the doctor is the expert in medicine. Patients have a responsibility to provide honest, complete, and accurate information; they make the final decisions about their own treatment; they are accountable for following through with agreed-upon plans. They must keep scheduled appointments and prepare for appointments with prioritized questions, and they must be encouraged to contact the doctor with any concerns, change in plans, or information about side effects.

The practitioner's job as an agent of healing in the treatment process is to provide the most effective treatment possible for the patient's condition. Clinicians have a responsibility to be open-minded and communicative, to listen carefully and ask all relevant questions, to be reasonably accessible, to keep their knowledge scientifically and clinically current, to maintain confidentiality and professionalism, and to acknowledge areas beyond their capabilities and refer for second opinions as necessary.

In our next and final chapter, we will present several case histories that exemplify how a more comprehensive approach to assessment and treatment can help the clinician improve outcomes for patients with depression. I am certain that you will have many wonderful experiences as you begin to use this new approach with your patients!

References

1. Corruble E, Falissard B, Gorwood P. Life events exposure before a treated major depressive episode depends on the number of past episodes. *Eur Psychiatry*. 2006;21:364-366.
2. Hedaya R. *Understanding Biological Psychiatry*. New York, NY: WW Norton and Co.; 1996.
3. Post RM. Transduction of psychosocial stress into the neurobiology of recurrent affective disorder. *Am J Psychiatry*. 1992;149:999-1010.
4. Oquendo MA, Currier D, Mann JJ. Prospective studies of suicidal behavior in major depressive and bipolar disorders: what is the evidence for predictive risk factors? *Acta Psychiatr Scand*. 2006;114:151-158.
5. Bibring E. The Mechanism of Depression. In: Greenacre P, ed. *Affective Disorders*. New York: International Universities Press; 1953.
6. Farabaugh A, Fava M, Mischoulon D, Sklarsky K, Petersen T, Alpert J. Relationships between major depressive disorder and comorbid anxiety and personality disorders. *Compr Psychiatry*. 2005;46:266-271.
7. Mulder RT. Depression and personality disorder. *Curr Psychiatry Rep*. 2004;6:51-57.
8. Gozansky WS, Lynn JS, Laudenslager ML, Kohrt WM. Salivary cortisol determined by enzyme immunoassay is preferable to serum total cortisol for assessment of dynamic hypothalamic—pituitary—adrenal axis activity. *Clin Endocrinol (Oxf)*. 2005;63:336-341.
9. Wong V, Yan T, Donald A, McLean M. Saliva and bloodspot cortisol: novel sampling methods to assess hydrocortisone replacement therapy in hypoadrenal patients. *Clin Endocrinol (Oxf)*. 2004;61:131-137.
10. Sabate JM, Jouet P, Harnois F, et al. high prevalence of small intestinal bacterial overgrowth in patients with morbid obesity: a contributor to severe hepatic steatosis. *Obes Surg*. 2008.
11. Hewison M, Gacad MA, Lemire J, Adams JS. Vitamin D as a cytokine and hematopoetic factor. *Rev Endocr Metab Disord*. 2001;2:217-227.
12. Hayes CE, Nashold FE, Spach KM, Pedersen LB. The immunological functions of the vitamin D endocrine system: *Cell Mol Biol (Noisy-le-grand)*. 2003;49:277-300.
13. Kilburn KH. Indoor mold exposure associated with neurobehavioral and pulmonary impairment: a preliminary report. *Arch Environ Health*. 2003;58:390-398.
14. Shenassa ED, Daskalakis C, Liebhaber A, Braubach M, Brown M. Dampness and mold in the home and depression: an examination of mold-related illness and perceived control of one's home as possible depression pathways. *Am J Public Health*. 2007;97:1893-1899.
15. Kilburn KH. Visual and neurobehavioral impairment associated with polychlorinated biphenyls. *Neurotoxicology*. 2000;21:489-499.
16. Bowler RM, Gysens S, Diamond E, Nakagawa S, Drezgic M, Roels HA. Manganese exposure: neuropsychological and neurological symptoms and effects in welders. *Neurotoxicology*. 2006;27:315-326.
17. Gandara BK, Leresche L, Mancl L. Patterns of salivary estradiol and progesterone across the menstrual cycle. *Ann N Y Acad Sci*. 2007;1098:446-450.
18. Stewart JW, Quitkin FM, McGrath PJ, Klein DF. Defining the boundaries of atypical depression: evidence from the HPA axis supports course of illness distinctions. *J Affect Disord*. 2005;86:161-167.
19. Rush AJ. The varied clinical presentations of major depressive disorder. *J Clin Psychiatry*. 2007;68 Suppl 8:4-10.
20. Wong ML, Kling MA, Munson PJ, et al. Pronounced and sustained central hypernoradrenergic function in major depression with melancholic features: relation to hypercortisolism and corticotropin-releasing hormone. *Proc Natl Acad Sci U S A*. 2000;97:325-330.

21. Gold PW, Gabry KE, Yasuda MR, Chrousos GP. Divergent endocrine abnormalities in melancholic and atypical depression: clinical and pathophysiologic implications. *Endocrinol Metab Clin North Am.* 2002;31:37-62, vi.

22. Swaab DF, Bao AM, Lucassen PJ. The stress system in the human brain in depression and neurodegeneration. *Ageing Res Rev.* 2005;4:141-194.

23. Matza LS, Revicki DA, Davidson JR, Stewart JW. Depression with atypical features in the National Comorbidity Survey: classification, description, and consequences. *Arch Gen Psychiatry.* 2003;60:817-826.

24. Tsigos C, Chrousos GP. Hypothalamic-pituitary-adrenal axis, neuroendocrine factors and stress. *J Psychosom Res.* 2002;53:865-871.

25. Gold PW, Chrousos GP. Organization of the stress system and its dysregulation in melancholic and atypical depression: high vs low CRH/NE states. *Mol Psychiatry.* 2002;7:254-275.

26. Schore AN. *Affect Regulation and the Repair of the Self.* New York, NY: W.W. Norton & Company, Inc.; 2003.

27. Fink GR, Markowitsch HJ, Reinkemeier M, Bruckbauer T, Kessler J, Heiss WD. Cerebral representation of one's own past: neural networks involved in autobiographical memory. *J Neurosci.* 1996;16:4275-4282.

28. Thase ME. New directions in the treatment of atypical depression. *J Clin Psychiatry.* 2007;67:e18.

29. Liebowitz MR, Quitkin FM, Stewart JW, et al. Antidepressant specificity in atypical depression. *Arch Gen Psychiatry.* 1988;45:129-137.

30. Quitkin FM, McGrath PJ, Stewart JW, et al. Atypical depression, panic attacks, and response to imipramine and phenelzine. A replication. *Arch Gen Psychiatry.* 1990;47:935-941.

31. Russo-Neustadt A, Beard RC, Cotman CW. Exercise, antidepressant medications, and enhanced brain derived neurotrophic factor expression. *Neuropsychopharmacology.* 1999;21:679-682.

32. Frank E, Kupfer DJ, Thase ME, et al. Two-year outcomes for interpersonal and social rhythm therapy in individuals with bipolar I disorder. *Arch Gen Psychiatry.* 2005;62:996-1004.

33. Lukaczer D. Oxidative stress and glycemic control. In: Jones DS, ed. *Textbook of Functional Medicine.* Gig Harbor, WA: Institute for Functional Medicine; 2005:526-541.

34. Bitar MS, Al-Saleh E, Al-Mulla F. Oxidative stress--mediated alterations in glucose dynamics in a genetic animal model of type II diabetes. *Life Sci.* 2005;77:2552-2573.

35. Bourre JM. Effects of nutrients (in food) on the structure and function of the nervous system: update on dietary requirements for brain. Part 1: micronutrients. *J Nutr Health Aging.* 2006;10:377-385.

36. Lukaczer D. The "4R" program. In: Jones DS, ed. *Textbook of Functional Medicine.* Gig Harbor, WA: Institute for Functional Medicine; 2005:462-479.

37. North CS, Hong BA, Alpers DH. Relationship of functional gastrointestinal disorders and psychiatric disorders: implications for treatment. *World J Gastroenterol.* 2007;13:2020-2027.

38. Roberts L, Wilson S, Singh S, Roalfe A, Greenfield S. Gut-directed hypnotherapy for irritable bowel syndrome: piloting a primary care-based randomised controlled trial. *Br J Gen Pract.* 2006;56:115-121.

39. Vlieger AM, Menko-Frankenhuis C, Wolfkamp SC, Tromp E, Benninga MA. Hypnotherapy for children with functional abdominal pain or irritable bowel syndrome: a randomized controlled trial. *Gastroenterology.* 2007;133:1430-1436.

40. Wilson S, Maddison T, Roberts L, Greenfield S, Singh S. Systematic review: the effectiveness of hypnotherapy in the management of irritable bowel syndrome. *Aliment Pharmacol Ther.* 2006;24:769-780.

41. Logan AC, Katzman M. Major depressive disorder: probiotics may be an adjuvant therapy. *Med Hypotheses.* 2005;64:533-538.

42. Majewski M, McCallum RW. Results of small intestinal bacterial overgrowth testing in irritable bowel syndrome patients: clinical profiles and effects of antibiotic trial. *Adv Med Sci.* 2007;52:139-142.

43. Paulionis L, Kane SL, Meckling KA. Vitamin status and cognitive function in a long-term care population. *BMC Geriatr.* 2005;5:16.

44. Bradford GS, Taylor CT. Omeprazole and vitamin B12 deficiency. *Ann Pharmacother.* 1999;33:641-643.

45. Alvarez JC, Cremniter D, Gluck N, et al. Low serum cholesterol in violent but not in non-violent suicide attempters. *Psychiatry Res.* 2000;95:103-108.

46. Placidi GP, Oquendo MA, Malone KM, Huang YY, Ellis SP, Mann JJ. Aggressivity, suicide attempts, and depression: relationship to cerebrospinal fluid monoamine metabolite levels. *Biol Psychiatry.* 2001;50:783-791.

47. Kessing LV, Sondergard L, Kvist K, Andersen PK. Suicide risk in patients treated with lithium. *Arch Gen Psychiatry.* 2005;62:860-866.

48. Sondergard L, Lopez AG, Andersen PK, Kessing LV. Mood-stabilizing pharmacological treatment in bipolar disorders and risk of suicide. *Bipolar Disord.* 2008;10:87-94.

49. Lopez-Leon S, Janssens AC, Gonzalez-Zuloeta Ladd AM, et al. Meta-analyses of genetic studies on major depressive disorder. *Mol Psychiatry.* 2007.

50. Kramer UM, Cunillera T, Camara E, et al. The impact of catechol-O-methyltransferase and dopamine D4 receptor genotypes on neurophysiological markers of performance monitoring. *J Neurosci.* 2007;27:14190-14198.

51. Gilbody S, Lewis S, Lightfoot T. Methylenetetrahydrofolate reductase (MTHFR) genetic polymorphisms and psychiatric disorders: a HuGE review. *Am J Epidemiol.* 2007;165:1-13.

52. Klerk M, Verhoef P, Clarke R, Blom HJ, Kok FJ, Schouten EG. MTHFR 677C-->T polymorphism and risk of coronary heart disease: a meta-analysis. *JAMA.* 2002;288:2023-2031.

53. Lin Z, Madras BK. Human genetics and pharmacology of neurotransmitter transporters. *Handb Exp Pharmacol.* 2006:327-371.

54. Isidori AM, Lenzi A. Ectopic ACTH syndrome. *Arq Bras Endocrinol Metabol.* 2007;51:1217-1225.

55. Schore A. Affect Regulation and the Repair of the Self: W. W. Norton; 2003.

56. Jeffries WM. *Safe Uses of Cortisol.* 3rd ed. Springfield, IL: Thomas Books; 2004.

57. Kronenberg HM, Melmed S, Polonsky KS, Larsen PR, eds. *Williams Textbook of Endocrinology.* 11th ed. Philadelphia, PA: Saunders; 2007.

58. Abraham G, Milev R, Stuart Lawson J. T3 augmentation of SSRI resistant depression. *J Affect Disord.* 2006;91:211-215.

59. Hollowell JG, Staehling NW, Flanders WD, et al. Serum TSH, T(4), and thyroid antibodies in the United States population (1988 to 1994): National Health and Nutrition Examination Survey (NHANES III). *J Clin Endocrinol Metab.* 2002;87:489-499.

60. Corruble E, Berlin I, Lemoine A, Hardy P. Should major depression with 'high normal' thyroid-stimulating hormone be treated preferentially with tricyclics? *Neuropsychobiology.* 2004;50:144-146.

61. Gitlin M, Altshuler LL, Frye MA, et al. Peripheral thyroid hormones and response to selective serotonin reuptake inhibitors. *J Psychiatry Neurosci.* 2004;29:383-386.

62. Maes M, Vandoolaeghe E, Neels H, et al. Lower serum zinc in major depression is a sensitive marker of treatment resistance and of the immune/inflammatory response in that illness. *Biol Psychiatry*. 1997;42:349-358.

63. Vasto S, Mocchegiani E, Malavolta M, et al. Zinc and inflammatory/immune response in aging. *Ann N Y Acad Sci*. 2007;1100:111-122.

64. Bedwal RS, Bahuguna A. Zinc, copper and selenium in reproduction. *Experientia*. 1994;50:626-640.

65. Gregoire AJ, Kumar R, Everitt B, Henderson AF, Studd JW. Transdermal oestrogen for treatment of severe postnatal depression. *Lancet*. 1996;347:930-933.

66. Smith RN, Studd JW, Zamblera D, Holland EF. A randomised comparison over 8 months of 100 micrograms and 200 micrograms twice weekly doses of transdermal oestradiol in the treatment of severe premenstrual syndrome. *Br J Obstet Gynaecol*. 1995;102:475-484.

67. Soares CN, Almeida OP, Joffe H, Cohen LS. Efficacy of estradiol for the treatment of depressive disorders in perimenopausal women: a double-blind, randomized, placebo-controlled trial. *Arch Gen Psychiatry*. 2001;58:529-534.

68. Gallagher P, Malik N, Newham J, Young A, Ferrier I, Mackin P. Antiglucocorticoid treatments for mood disorders. *Cochrane Database Syst Rev*. 2008:CD005168.

69. Rabkin JG, McElhiney MC, Rabkin R, McGrath PJ, Ferrando SJ. Placebo-controlled trial of dehydroepiandrosterone (DHEA) for treatment of nonmajor depression in patients with HIV/AIDS. *Am J Psychiatry*. 2006;163:59-66.

70. Schmidt PJ, Daly RC, Bloch M, et al. Dehydroepiandrosterone monotherapy in midlife-onset major and minor depression. *Arch Gen Psychiatry*. 2005;62:154-162.

71. McCann SE, Wactawski-Wende J, Kufel K, et al. Changes in 2-hydroxyestrone and 16alpha-hydroxyestrone metabolism with flaxseed consumption: modification by COMT and CYP1B1 genotype. *Cancer Epidemiol Biomarkers Prev*. 2007;16:256-262.

72. Weng JR, Tsai CH, Kulp SK, Chen CS. Indole-3-carbinol as a chemopreventive and anti-cancer agent. *Cancer Lett*. 2008.

73. Campbell KL, Westerlind KC, Harber VJ, Friedenreich CM, Courneya KS. Associations between aerobic fitness and estrogen metabolites in premenopausal women. *Med Sci Sports Exerc*. 2005;37:585-592.

74. Campbell KL, Westerlind KC, Harber VJ, Bell GJ, Mackey JR, Courneya KS. Effects of aerobic exercise training on estrogen metabolism in premenopausal women: a randomized controlled trial. *Cancer Epidemiol Biomarkers Prev*. 2007;16:731-739.

75. Larsson SC, Kumlin M, Ingelman-Sundberg M, Wolk A. Dietary long-chain n-3 fatty acids for the prevention of cancer: a review of potential mechanisms. *Am J Clin Nutr*. 2004;79:935-945.

76. Schatzberg AF, Nemeroff CB. *The American Psychiatric Publishing Textbook of Psychopharmacology*. 2nd ed. Washington, DC: American Psychiatric Publishing; 1998.

77. Jurcic J, Pereira JA, Kavanaugh D. St John's wort versus paroxetine for depression. *Can Fam Physician*. 2007;53:1511-1513.

78. Kasper S, Gastpar M, Muller WE, et al. Efficacy of St. John's wort extract WS 5570 in acute treatment of mild depression: a reanalysis of data from controlled clinical trials. *Eur Arch Psychiatry Clin Neurosci*. 2008;258:59-63.

79. van der Watt G, Laugharne J, Janca A. Complementary and alternative medicine in the treatment of anxiety and depression. *Curr Opin Psychiatry*. 2008;21:37-42.

80. Coppen A, Bailey J. Enhancement of the antidepressant action of fluoxetine by folic acid: a randomised, placebo controlled trial. *J Affect Disord*. 2000;60:121-130.

81. Gilbody S, Lightfoot T, Sheldon T. Is low folate a risk factor for depression? A meta-analysis and exploration of heterogeneity. *J Epidemiol Community Health*. 2007;61:631-637.

Chapter 8

Clinical Cases

Case History — Carl

Carl, a 59-year-old, married, international policy analyst, reported a history of severe melancholic depression, beginning at age 43. He recovered substantially but was left with a waxing and waning, low-grade depression (dysthymia). At 57, he was father to 6 children, enmeshed in a failing marriage, and had started a new business venture in China. In the year before we first met, he was traveling back and forth between the United States and China 3 times per month, on average.

The initial evaluation and workup revealed a man who was alienated from his wife, succeeding in his business, and falling into fits of depression and irritability. His nutrition was poor, he was episodically drinking to induce sleep, he was not exercising, and his church attendance, while reasonably regular, was devoid of spirit. A review of his personal history strongly suggested that the presentation of a melancholic depression out of the blue at age 43 was probably inaccurate. His personal history revealed a markedly unstable mother with very high performance demands and unpredictable anger, as well as social bullying and alienation from the dominant community culture. In all likelihood, this early misattunement and emotional abuse helped set the stage for his affective disorder; for the most part (except for the index episode at age 43), his disorder took the form of an atypical, rejection-sensitive, hypocortisolemic, hyponoradrenergic depression.

Metabolically, he had a variety of nutrient deficiencies, and his adrenal function was impaired. His dehydroepiandrosterone (DHEA) was significantly below normal, and his 24-hour urinary catecholamines (dopamine and epinephrine) were in the lowest percentiles of the normal range.

At the initial visit, he was on a low dose of an antidepressant and a benzodiazepine. Via exercise, a change in diet, meditation, therapy (IPT, geared toward helping him function better as a husband), and a 90% reduction in his travel, he was stabilized and significantly improved. His family life settled down, and his marriage reached a higher level of satisfaction than it had since the first onset of his depression at age 43. However, he continued to have periodic descents into depression lasting up to 3 weeks. After 2 years of treatment, his adrenal stress index revealed a very low cortisol on 3 separate occasions (in the face of a normal adrenocorticotrophic hormone [ACTH] stimulation test). A trial of oral hydrocortisone (10 mg on waking, 5 mg at 11 AM, and 5 mg at 3 PM) made a remarkable difference, eliminating 80% of his remaining depression and normalizing his ability to cope with stress.

Case History — Benjamin

In June 1985, Benjamin sat in the corner seat of my waiting room, feeling distraught and humiliated. Recently released after 3 weeks of hospitalization on the psychiatry ward, this rejection-sensitive young man was still highly anxious, experiencing panic, hopelessness, and suicidal ideation. His pain was poorly disguised by a thin veneer of humor. Using a combination of individual (cognitive-behavioral) and group therapies and phenelzine (an MAO inhibitor) over 5 years, he gradually came to live a full life, and his visits to me were reduced to a biannual event, when I would catch up with his news and enjoy his excellent sense of humor. In 1989, I switched Benjamin over to fluoxetine (Prozac®), which lacked the MAO-associated risk of causing a hypertensive crisis. Benjamin did quite well; he eventually married and had 3 children.

With the passage of time, Benjamin's wife, stressed by the maternal role (which her own mother had abdicated), developed fibromyalgia. His parents' health and finances deteriorated. As the breadwinner of his own family and only surviving child to his parents, his stress level rose significantly. In August 1999, Benjamin came for a visit before his usual 6-month checkup. Fourteen years after his first panic and depression, he was now having a recurrence of the panic attacks, usually before his singing performances. He was tormented by the recurring thought that he was on an inevitable downhill slide that would result in his being sent back to the hospital. He was convinced that he needed to change his medication to sertraline (Zoloft®). "I think it's Prozac poop-out," he said.

Knowing that it was important to deal directly with the negative thought and the preoccupation, I asked Benjamin what basis he had for thinking this, and we explored his logic. I asked him whether there were any other ways of looking at the situation. I reassured him that what he feared would not happen and explained the reasons why. I pointed out that panic can easily be treated with a short-acting benzodiazepine while searching for the cause of increased symptoms, and I suggested that we could increase the frequency of our contact as needed, rather than use the hospital. He now had a relationship with a psychiatrist he trusted and who cared about him, whereas that was not the case 15 years earlier.

> **Clinical Pearl:**
>
> In depression, regardless of the cause (e.g., metabolic, nutritional, social), distortions in thinking (e.g., catastrophizing or all-or-nothing attitudes) are usually present. Selective attention to these distorted thoughts is the norm for depressed patients. One aspect of treatment is identifying these thoughts, elucidating the nature of the distortion, and testing the logic behind the automatic assumption. For a full description of these distortions, read *Cognitive Therapy of Depression* by Aaron Beck et al[1] or *Feeling Good* by David Burns.[2]

Untended, this catastrophic fear was causing Benjamin to experience anticipatory anxiety (activating his dorsal raphé nucleus), which was priming his limbic system for panic (locus coeruleus) and generating a feed-forward cycle via the amygdala and locus coeruleus that was developing into full-fledged panic. The hypothalamic-pituitary-adrenal (HPA) axis activation with a positive feedback loop could have become a self-fulfilling prophecy.

Having addressed these issues, I then explained to Benjamin that "Prozac poop-out" (the commonly held idea that antidepressants often stop working after a while) is not a concept that is supported by the evidence. If a person with unipolar depression is fully responding to an antidepressant in an essentially stable manner for several months or more and then relapses, it is incumbent on the practitioner to search for other factors that are now overriding the medication (assuming adherence to the medication), such as psychosocial changes and stressors, as well as any other aspect of the Functional Medicine Matrix Model.

At this point, I decided that in order to approach the situation with a fresh perspective, I would evaluate Benjamin as if he were a new patient. I would do my best to leave no stone unturned, no assumption unchallenged. I started with the psychosocial stressors (being a parent, having an ill wife and parents, being the sole breadwinner) and delved into the nature of how these stressors had changed his life and how he had adapted to the changes.

Benjamin had taken a partial detour from his own career in order to manage his parents' finances, control his mother's spending, and sell his father's business. When the day was done, he would come home to his ill wife and do most of the housework. Having little support, Benjamin began to cope by stress eating. He gained weight and began to experience indigestion, intermittent nausea, and lower gastrointestinal cramping. His family doctor, concerned about gastroesophageal reflux and perhaps an ulcer, had placed him on omeprazole (Prilosec®). Benjamin had noticed a significant improvement in his digestion and had been on the drug for 5 years before his present panic attacks and depression recurred. The recurrence of panic shook his confidence, and he felt that he was once again losing control of his life and his mind. He began using alprazolam (Xanax®) before his performances.

Knowing that omeprazole can inhibit vitamin B12 absorption (by inhibiting the gastric parietal cells that produce intrinsic factor, which is necessary for B12 absorption), I eventually convinced Benjamin that he should be worked up for a B12 deficiency secondary to the omeprazole. Despite his distress, he was quite resistant to this idea. Martin Seligman's learned helplessness model of depression demonstrates that, despite their pain, some depressed individuals actively resist help.[3] The neurophysiology of mood disorders suggests that a certain part of the prefrontal cortex (the ventromedial PFC), whose function is to accurately predict or anticipate rewarding experiences and pleasure or painful consequences, has reduced activity in depression.[4]

The detection of B12 deficiency is difficult. One can look for a macrocytic anemia, low serum B12 levels, or high levels of methylmalonic acid. However, several studies indicate that these tests are often falsely normal when tested against the gold standard Schilling test[5] (no longer available) or the more recently studied holotranscobalamin.[6, 7]

When Benjamin finally agreed to the workup, he turned out to have a B12 deficiency, an iron deficiency, and some unidentified infectious/inflammatory condition. His methylmalonic acid and complete blood count (CBC) were within normal limits, although his mean corpuscular volume (MCV) was trending to the lower limit of normal (84.1 µm, normal = 80–100), and his serum iron was low (29 µg/dL, normal = 40–155). These trends suggested to me that a macrocytic anemia could have been developing, but if so, it was certainly obscured by the low iron (a result of gastrointestinal bleeding creating a microcytic tendency). The only frankly abnormal test of B12 status was a functional intracellular assay of B12 function, which was markedly low (9%, normal > 15%).

Because Benjamin also complained of indigestion, bloating, constipation, and gassiness, I evaluated him for bacterial overgrowth of the small intestine (normal), which can impair nutrient absorption. An IgG panel for delayed food sensitivities revealed many food sensitivities (29), and a digestive stool analysis revealed borderline elevation in pH (consistent with his use of omeprazole), highly elevated (4+) *Candida* overgrowth, rare to moderate white blood cells (suggestive of infection or an inflammatory process such as ulcerative colitis), rare red blood cells, and *Klebsiella* (+3). As a result of the testing, Benjamin was placed on a 4R program[i] (which included the elimination of food sensitivities and an anti-*Candida* regimen), a dysglycemia program (due to a HgA1C of 6.2), an iron supplement, and B12 (injectable) 1000 µg 3 times per week for 1 month, then once per week for 2 months (after which he was switched to sublingual). Clinical signs and symptoms also suggested sleep apnea; however, he refused to do a sleep study, so he was instructed to use a "snore ball" (2 tennis balls sewn into the back of a T-shirt to prevent him from sleeping on his back). Finally, he began a moderate exercise program, which he could do at work. In the meantime, his internist evaluated him for gallbladder disease, which turned up negative.

Four months after starting this regimen, Benjamin returned to the office and stated, "The nausea is almost totally gone. The anxiety is 80% better. I am less tired and more energetic since starting the B12." He now told me that before his performances, he had been feeling a flu-like syndrome including achiness, feverishness, lethargy, and vomiting or gagging. His use of alprazolam was now reduced to once per 2 weeks, and he was beginning to believe that "I won't be addicted to Xanax." Six months later, after being off the injectable B12 for a few months, he reported, "The sublingual B12 isn't working. The nausea came back, so I restarted the B12 injections. After 3 weeks on the injectable

---

[i] The 4R program is described in detail in the *Textbook of Functional Medicine*, pg. 462-468; it is a program of gut restoration that involves four steps: Remove, Replace, Reinoculate, and Repair.

B12, I am almost back to normal." Before the relapse, he had been running 2 miles three times per week. His internist had changed him to pantoprazole (Protonix®) a few months earlier, but we had never changed the fluoxetine. About 1 year after our initial investigations began, he reported that he had recently done "8 shows in 1 week and hadn't needed an alprazolam in 2–3 months… B12 seems to be the key to the nausea." Eventually Benjamin did a sleep study, which revealed sleep apnea. He began to use CPAP, which ended his snoring and improved his energy.

Over the ensuing 3 years, Benjamin worked with his wife (who was at one point threatening separation) in couple's therapy and followed his diet and exercise regimen intermittently, usually for several months at a time. He lost 10–15 lbs. He continued on pantoprazole until he had surgery for gastroesophageal reflux, which allowed him to eliminate the pantoprazole. His marriage improved, and his overall health was better. Throughout this process, it was not necessary to change his antidepressant; he was able to discontinue his use of alprazolam, and he did not suffer a significant episode of depression.

There are many factors operative in this case, illustrating that intervention in multiple aspects of the Functional Medicine Matrix was critical in Benjamin's achieving an overall improvement in his health, using less medication, and eliminating significant depression and anxiety. The effects of Benjamin's B12 deficiency manifested themselves first in his weakest system—his nervous system. With the introduction of B12 injections, Benjamin's panic (manifested by a feeling of nausea) and depression cleared completely. He has been without panic or depression since then (with 7 years of follow-up).

Case History — Heather

Heather was a 38-year-old, divorced and remarried, successful event planner, who was on lithium carbonate 600 mg/d, fexofenadine (Allegra®), Triamcinolone (Nasacort®), albuterol, and montelukast (Singulair®) at the time of her initial visit with me. Over the preceding 8 years, she had been on multiple antidepressants that had often caused agitation (which is suggestive of either a temporal lobe dysfunction or a bipolar tendency), mood stabilizers (she was either noncompliant with these or she "couldn't tolerate them"), and antipsychotics ("couldn't tolerate"). Her presenting concerns were:

- "I am bipolar and have had depression since 1998. My moods are erratic, with 5-day cycles—they used to be every 6 months to a year. I don't think the lithium helps."
- "I have anxiety when I am hypomanic."

She had multiple other physical complaints:

- Premenstrual migraines, chronic sinusitis, fatigue, seasonal depression, irritability, and insomnia
- Signs and symptoms of hypothyroidism, adrenal fatigue, and hypoglycemia
- Symptoms consistent with chronic fatigue immune deficiency syndrome (CFIDS)
- A previous diagnosis of irritable bowel syndrome, with numerous gastrointestinal complaints (frequent diarrhea, bloating, belching, flatulence)

Heather came to me because she and her new husband wanted to have a child together but were concerned that the lithium would put the baby at risk. Despite her medication, she was moderately depressed (Beck Depression Inventory was 27, normal < 10), and her score on the Medical Symptoms Questionnaire (form included in the Appendix) was markedly elevated at 121. Her Beck Anxiety Inventory was 22 (normal < 10). Feeling stuck, she and her husband were at a loss as to what to do.

The assessment of what medications are safe to use during pregnancy generally involves a risk-benefit analysis. Together with the patient, the healthcare provider must balance the known and unknown risks of teratogenicity with the risk of depression during pregnancy and especially in the postpartum period. Consequently, I took a very careful history and decided that if Heather did indeed have bipolar disorder, it was certainly mild. I was more convinced that she had unipolar depression with a temporal lobe dysregulation—she acknowledged spontaneous anxiety without a cognitive or environmental stimulus; she had experienced brief periods of time with lack of awareness, olfactory sensitivity if not hallucinations, significant irritability, macropsia, micropsia, frequent déjà vu and jamais vu episodes, and visual illusions; and she had difficulty expressing herself verbally and finding words. Before her menses, she would often have severe migraines with facial paresthesia and difficulty with articulation. She reported having taken valproic acid (Depakote®) for 5 days, which helped.

Given the multiple indications of hormonal, digestive, and immune/inflammatory dysregulation in the history, it was a reasonable hypothesis that improving the function of these systems would have a positive effect on her mood stability. Disturbances in these systems can interfere with brain function in innumerable ways, as has been documented elsewhere in this monograph.

Heather's physical exam was remarkable for dry skin, mild pedal edema, mild thyromegaly bilaterally, and mild hirsutism. We evaluated her nutritional, hormonal, detoxification, gastrointestinal, and immune function. This workup generated the following findings:

- **Nutritional** — Multiple nutritional deficiencies were detected. Magnesium and zinc were at the lowest limit of normal; vitamin B12, pantothenic acid, and 25-hydroxy vitamin D3 were also low. Essential and conditionally essential amino acids were low, including tryptophan, methionine, valine, leucine, isoleucine, tyrosine, glycine, and serine; gamma-aminobutyric acid (GABA) was at the upper limit of normal. Phosphoethanolamine (PE) was markedly elevated (51 mmol/L, normal < 30). According to Bralley and Lord,[8] high PE may indicate functional impairment of acetylcholine synthesis, as PE is methylated with S-adenosylmethionine (SAMe) in this process. Functional vitamin B12 or folate deficiency or disordered methionine metabolism (i.e., inhibition of methyl group transfer) may account for high PE levels. Low glycine, low serine, and high GABA suggest difficulty producing acetylcholine, as well. Individuals with high PE may experience depression or other effects on brain function because GABA binding is inhibited by PE.
- **Detoxification** — Glutathione conjugation was impaired (4.6%, normal = 5.6% to 11.4%).
- **Inflammation** — There was marked elevation of free radical markers consistent with inflammation (2,3-dihydroxybenzoic acid, urine peroxides, catechol).
- **Immune** — There was reduced natural killer (NK) cell activity (10.1 LUs, normal = 20–50) and evidence of *Mycoplasma* and Epstein-Barr virus infection in the past. There were 7 food sensitivities, including brewer's and baker's yeasts.
- **Endocrine** — The 2-hour insulin/glucose tolerance test was normal. TSH was elevated (3.5 μIU/mL, normal = 0.4–3.0) with midrange free T3, free T4, and reverse T3. Very mild adrenal insufficiency was noted (subnormal noon salivary cortisol and borderline low DHEA of 3μmol/L, normal = 3–1). Melatonin was normal.
- **Gastrointestinal** — A digestive stool analysis revealed "many *Blastocystis hominis* (parasite), "few red blood cells," and borderline low pancreatic elastase (351 μg/g, optimal range ≥ 500, low ≤ 201), suggestive of impaired digestive enzyme production. Her stool pH was on the high side of optimal (7.2, normal = 6.1–7.9)

Based on the above findings, we treated the gastrointestinal infection, instituted a 4R program, followed the adrenal and thyroid closely, replenished the deficient nutrients, and tapered the lithium. Heather also began a mild exercise program. Exercise is known to have antidepressant effects equal to medication in mild and moderate depression in many individuals (see Chapters 6 and 7). It increases levels of brain-derived neurotrophic factor (BDNF), a growth factor also stimulated by antidepressant medications. Therefore, an exercise regimen is an important aspect of the treatment of depression, assuming there are no contraindications. It should be instituted in a graded fashion, combining stretching, weight-bearing, and aerobic activities.

A supplement (ImmPower™, a mushroom extract, 2 capsules three times per day for 1 month) was used to boost her NK cell activity into the normal range (47 LUs), thereby improving her ability to fight viruses and bacteria. (Once an effective supplement is found for NK cell activity, it is continued indefinitely). This is relevant to the treatment of mood disorders, since cytokines and immune activation are known to increase depressed mood, reduce cognitive ability, and increase anxiety. (See Chapter 6, *Mechanisms and Interconnections within the Functional Medicine Matrix Model*.) With fewer infections, one of Heather's triggers for mood instability was removed.

The *Blastocystis* was stubborn and required the sequential use of tinidazole (500 mg twice per day for 14 days), metronidazole (750 mg three times per day for 10 days), and paromomycin sulfate (250 mg four times per day for 21 days), concurrent with nystatin (oral suspension 100,000 units/mL, 1 teaspoon four times per day between meals), probiotics, and a natural antiparasitic agent (Para-Gard®). The literature is divided on whether *Blastocystis* does indeed cause clinical symptoms.[9, 10] We chose to treat it as part of a comprehensive 4R program since Heather had so many gastrointestinal symptoms (with few other possible explanations) and probable malabsorption of nutrients, which can affect mood directly via neurotransmitter depletion and indirectly via increased susceptibility to infection and free radical injury.

> **Clinical Pearl:**
>
> Sometimes patients and physicians prefer to treat one variable at a time in the hope that the cause of the problem can thus be identified. In my experience with complex, chronic illness, it is rarely possible to determine a single cause. Linear thinking can slow down the pace of recovery and often cannot differentiate whether a specific intervention is necessary but not sufficient for recovery. Treating all identified variables when possible is most likely to improve outcomes.

Early in the treatment, Heather failed to take the probiotics and developed an oral *Candida* infection, despite clear instructions and a very good working relationship between us. This underlines the need to pay serious attention to compliance during treatment. Noncompliance is more common than most practitioners think. According to a study by Trivedi,[11] "...only 25% to 50% of patients with major depressive disorder adhere to their antidepressant regimen for the length of time recommended by depression guidelines..." In this case, I discussed both the reasons for her not following instructions ("I didn't think I needed the probiotics") and the idea of working in a partnership with me ("You know your life and body best, but I know medicine best. Together we can make a very effective team. If I suggest something you are not comfortable with, let me know").

Ultimately, the parasite was eradicated (the second stool test, 6 weeks after the first, showed moderate *Blastocystis*; however, the parasite was eliminated by the third stool test approximately 3 months later), and essentially all of Heather's gastrointestinal complaints cleared with the 4R program. Gradually, her immune function improved ("I haven't gotten sick"), and she "cut way back" on her asthma and allergy medications without any problems. Notably, Heather went through the winter without any significant seasonal depression and has been medication free for the past 15 months without any significant mood disturbance. "The biggest thing is that I am off meds. I would take them and have to deal with all these side effects. It's a huge win for me. I feel more in control of what's going on with me. I appreciate that you listen to me."

The changes on Heather's amino acid analysis revealed a normalization of most of the amino acids, although her tryptophan level remained low despite twice daily supplementation with a personalized, powdered, free-form amino acid formula (with 250 mg additional tyrosine), indicating a likely failure of absorption due to competition for transport with other neutral amino acids.[12] Importantly, her level of PE was reduced from 51 to 11 mmol/L, suggesting normalization of the metabolic pathways involving acetylcholine production.

Heather's immune function and migraines are markedly better. Her sinusitis continues to be an occasional problem, but she is able to use a supplement (echinacea) to which she responds right away ("I haven't been sick in quite some time"). A home assessment for mold (her basement flooded on 2 occasions) resulted in mold remediation, which may have helped, as well. While Heather still experiences episodic fatigue, she reports (and her husband confirms) that she is much better. At the time of this writing, Heather has been trying to get pregnant for 5 months.

The long-term management of Heather's mood disorder is not certain. The decision to discontinue medication use is not to be taken lightly, particularly in those with a history of recurrent depression and suicidal ideation or attempts with marked role impairment. Heather's decision was based on her desire to become pregnant, the mild nature of the depression, and the finding of multiple metabolic factors that were very likely affecting her mood stability. A study by Frank[13] looked at 128 people with recurrent unipolar depression over a 3-year period. They were divided into 5 groups: interpersonal therapy with and without drug placebo, placebo alone, interpersonal therapy with medication, medication clinic and placebo, and medication clinic with active medication. The study indicates a high relapse rate over a 3-year period with placebo treatment (approximately 85%) and only a 20% relapse rate with medication. At 1 year, the relapse rate for medication clinic and placebo treatment was almost 80%. This study did not assess other variables, such as those discussed in this monograph; however, it does indicate the chronic nature of depression. It also supports the probability that Heather's improvement is not a placebo response, since her chance of relapse on placebo treatment was almost 80% within the first year. Of course, eliminating a parasite, providing nutritional support, improving immune regulation, and increasing exercise are not placebo treatments. While it is prudent to keep open the possibility that Heather may need medication again, it seems clear that the advanced paradigm presented in this monograph has enabled her to improve her health in many ways, including significantly improving her mood stability without medication and allowing the possibility of having a child without the risk of teratogenicity.

Case History — Mark

Mark was a 64-year-old obese attorney in a high-powered law firm. He was approaching retirement and had come back to see me after a 10-year hiatus, complaining of depression and nearly intolerable anxiety. A thorough evaluation revealed:

- Nutritional abnormalities:
    - Markedly low 25-hydroxy vitamin D (9 ng/mL, normal = 20–100)
    - Depleted levels of red blood cell omega-3 essential fatty acids (alpha-linolenic acid at 0.11%, normal = 0.28%; eicosapentaenoic acid at 0.40%, normal = 0.43%), elevated docosahexaenoic acid at 4.23% (normal = 3.46%), and slightly elevated omega-6 essential fatty acids (32.86%, normal = 31.32%)
    - Niacin deficiency determined by functional intracellular assay (62%, normal > 81%)
    - Coenzyme Q10 deficiency (0.6 mg/L, normal = 0.8–1.5)
    - Vitamin E deficiency (10.7 mg/L, normal = 12.0–50)
    - Beta-carotene deficiency (< 0.2 mg/L, normal = 0.4–3.5) and vitamin A (0.6 mg/L, normal= 0.5–1.2)
- *Blastocystis hominis* (He was an international traveler in his legal capacity, which increased his risk for exposure to parasites)
- 30 IgG food sensitivities
- Obstructive sleep apnea syndrome with moderate oxygen desaturation (a low of 87%, 93% at baseline) and periodic leg movements during sleep (periodic leg movement index of 17 per hour); he was unable to tolerate CPAP
- Hormones:
    - DHEA markedly subnormal at 87 ng/dL (normal = 180–1250)
    - Markedly elevated salivary cortisol throughout the day, but quite low on waking (8 AM, 5 nmol, normal = 13–24; 11 AM, 20 nmol, normal 5–10; 4 PM, 9 nmol, normal = 3–8; 11 PM, 6 nmol, normal 1–4)
- Elevated 24-hour urinary dopamine (540 µg; normal = 52–480)
- Elevated PSA (9.3 ng/mL, normal = 0.0–4.0) (which led to a subsequent diagnosis of prostate cancer)
- Genetics:
    - Homozygous (++) for COMT V158M polymorphism
    - CYP 450 1B1 polymorphism

While there are many interesting aspects to this case, the genetic polymorphisms affected both the treatment of Mark's anxiety and his development of prostate cancer, so those are the elements we will discuss here. Catechol-O-methyl transferase is an enzyme present in the synaptic cleft. It degrades catecholamines such as dopamine, noradrenalin, and estrogens using SAMe as a carbon donor. People who have the COMT polymorphism produce an enzyme that is slow in degrading these catecholamines. "COMT, the major enzyme determining cortical dopamine flux, has a common functional polymorphism (val[158]met) that affects prefrontal function and working memory capacity and has also been associated with anxiety and emotional dysregulation."[14] There is significant evidence that this single nucleotide polymorphism (SNP) is related to increased risk for a variety of psychiatric problems including ADD, alcoholism, mood disorders, schizophrenia, and "inflexible processing of affective stimuli."[14] In addition, this SNP has been identified as a risk factor for prostate cancer via its effect on estrogen metabolism.[15] Also of interest is the evidence that DHEA (remember, Mark's was low—probably as a result of his chronic stress) probably inhibits the hepatic expression and activity of the carcinogen-activating enzyme CYP 1B1 *in vivo*.[16] We can only speculate on the possible link between his chronic stress (which reduced levels of the protective DHEA) and his prostate cancer, but there is certainly evidence suggestive of the connection.

Mark's 2 SNPs mean that he will always have higher levels of catecholamines and estrogens synaptically and perhaps systemically. We cannot be certain whether his postsynaptic metabotropic (G-protein linked) receptors and second and third messengers (intracellularly) were able to adapt and compensate for this overstimulation (although his lifelong history of anxiety would argue that such downregulation, if it did occur, was insufficient). But we can be certain of one thing: Mark's fronto-limbic circuitry was dysregulated from an early age. The genetic finding implied that to help him with his mood and anxiety, we might do best to improve COMT activity and reduce catecholamine levels (e.g. dopamine and norepinephrine, which can be associated with anxiety), rather than the more traditional GABAergic (e.g., benzodiazepine) or antidepressant/anti-anxiety (e.g., venlafaxine) approaches.

Treatment choices to consider, based on the genetic testing, included SAMe and folic acid (necessary precursor for SAMe) to maximize activity of the COMT enzyme by providing the methyl donor it requires for activity. Alternatively, we could consider a dopamine blocker (the antipsychotic medications inhibit or block dopamine receptors in all four of the major dopamine pathways in the brain). Mark wanted quick relief, so he elected to use a dopamine blocker, quetiapine (Seroquel®). Normally, this is not used for anxiety or depression; rather, it is used for individuals with a psychotic disorder or those in a manic phase, since there are significant and potentially serious side effects, including tardive dyskinesia, insulin resistance, and induction of type 2 diabetes. However, the genetics (and the elevated dopamine in the 24-hour urine) suggested this might be an appropriate short-term approach. Mark responded immediately, stating, "I cannot recall being so free of anxiety at any time in my life!" This example of how genetics can influence treatment choices reinforces the importance of considering all aspects of the patient and tailoring treatments that can take into account biochemical individuality.

Another genetic influence to consider in the treatment of affective disorders is the methylenetetrahydrofolate reductase (MTHFR) SNP, as it has significant effects on folic acid metabolism, which is associated with affective disorder and its treatment. A normal enzyme helps activate folate to 5-methyltetrahydrofolate, which is critical in the methylation process, ubiquitous in the central nervous system (and the rest of the body), and necessary for neurotransmitter homeostasis. Folic acid supplementation has been shown to enhance the effectiveness of antidepressant medication, to reduce side effects of medication, and even to be effective as an antidepressant alone, albeit in very high doses. (For more on folic acid and MTHFR, see Chapters 6 and 7.)

As a side note, Mark had excessive exposure to estrogen due to both the COMT and the CYP 450 1B1 SNPs. CYP 450 1B1 controls an enzymatic reaction that catalyzes the methylation of catecholestrogens (2- or 4 hydroxyestrogens) to 2- or 4 methoxy-estrogens, as well as the production of 4-hydroxyestrogens from estrogen.[17] Estrogen has been implicated in the development of prostate cancer.[18] It is certainly possible that these 2 genes, in combination with other factors such as diet and stress, increased his risk for prostate cancer.

Case History — Tamika

Tamika, a 48-year-old, married, African-American professional, came to me with a diagnosis of bipolar disorder. She had been hospitalized with manic episodes on 3 occasions and with severe depression once. She had seen numerous psychiatrists and psychopharmacologists over the years, never achieving stability in the improvement of her mood disorder for more than a few months since the age of 24. With minor adjustments of her medication and improved nutrition and hormone function (thyroid, melatonin), Tamika had been stable and free of depression and mania for nearly 5 years.

Initially, she had been quite compliant with her medication, supplements, diet (geared to correct her insulin resistance and food sensitivities), and exercise regimen. Her teenage son and daughter, who had assumed a parental role in the home, were very pleased with their mother's stability. However, as time went on, Tamika began to resent the treatment. For 2 years, I approached Tamika's resentment and growing noncompliance from a logical, cognitive point of view. Our conversations went something like this:

RH: "How are you doing, Tamika, with your program?"

T: "Well, I'm OK. But I know I should be doing better."

RH: "What do you mean?"

T: "Well, I miss my medication often. I go to sleep late. I wake up late and get to work late. I am not eating properly, and I often miss my exercise and vitamins."

RH: "What happens? Why do you miss your medication?"

T: "Well, I don't know. I see them right in front of me, but I forget to take them."

RH: "Why don't you try putting them on the dinner table?"

T: "That's a good idea."

> **Clinical Pearl:**
>
> Unconscious factors are quite often at the base of so-called noncompliance or nonadherence. Not all patients are capable of uncovering these hidden complexes of behavior, as Carl Jung termed them, but many are. If the clinician can learn to address the underlying history of the behaviors, which generally stem from painful experiences, the success of the treatment can be greatly enhanced.

Yet sure enough, the next visit would produce a Tamika with greater shame and frustration, but unimproved compliance. No matter what plan we came up with (e.g., e-mailing me with her sleep and medication schedule daily), no matter how logical it was, no matter how well it seemed to solve the apparent problem, it never worked.

We rode this not-so-merry-go-round for 2 years. Then one day, I was able to step out of the linear "Dr. Fix-it" mode. I became interested in what was behind this logic- and willpower-defying process. I asked Tamika about her family history around doctors and medication. This opened the floodgates, revealing a history in which her abusive stepfather shamed her mother for taking medication for a "white man's disease" (depression). Her former husband had echoed that cultural belief. Her irregularity around basic functions such as meals and sleep was strongly influenced by a childhood history of erratic mealtimes and irregular schedules. When this pattern became clear, Tamika was appalled at the idea that her abusive stepfather and former husband were apparently, albeit unconsciously, still controlling her life choices every time she looked at her vitamins and medications or otherwise attempted to stick with her treatment plan. She left the office deeply disturbed. At the next visit 1 month later, Tamika was monitoring her compliance on paper ("something I could *never, ever* have done before"). She realized that her resentment of the most successful treatment she had ever had was based on a belief that I, like her stepfather and former husband, was in control of her life; for a while, she felt that I had actually saved her life. When, via a writing workshop, she realized that I did not save her life and that it was she who was making the choices, she began to be liberated. Her compliance has gradually grown, as we have explored the unconscious foundations of her resistance to treatment. As she has moved into ownership of her life and her self-care, she has become vibrant and radiant, as well as more active in her life.

References

1. Beck AT, Rush AJ, Shaw BF, Emery G. *Cognitive Therapy of Depression*. New York, NY: The Guilford Press; 1979.
2. Burns DD. *Feeling Good*. New York, NY: Avon Books; 1999.
3. Seligman MEP. *Helplessness: On Depression, Development, and Death*. San Francisco: Freeman; 1975.
4. Johnstone T, van Reekum CM, Urry HL, Kalin NH, Davidson RJ. Failure to regulate: counterproductive recruitment of top-down prefrontal-subcortical circuitry in major depression. *J Neurosci*. 2007;27:8877-8884.
5. Lindenbaum J, Healton EB, Savage DG, et al. Neuropsychiatric disorders caused by cobalamin deficiency in the absence of anemia or macrocytosis. *N Engl J Med*. 1988;318:1720-1728.
6. Herrmann W, Obeid R, Schorr H, Geisel J. Functional vitamin B12 deficiency and determination of holotranscobalamin in populations at risk. *Clin Chem Lab Med*. 2003;41:1478-1488.
7. Herrmann W, Obeid R, Schorr H, Geisel J. The usefulness of holotranscobalamin in predicting vitamin B12 status in different clinical settings. *Curr Drug Metab*. 2005;6:47-53.
8. Bralley J, Lord R. *Laboratory Evaluations in Molecular Medicine*. Norcross, GA: The Institute for Advances in Molecular Medicine; 2001.
9. Sun T, Katz S, Tanenbaum B, Schenone C. Questionable clinical significance of Blastocystis hominis infection. *Am J Gastroenterol*. 1989;84:1543-1547.
10. Zdero M, Cabrera G, Ponce de Leon P, Nocito I, Echenique C. [Parasitosis in an adult population with chronic gastrointestinal disorders]. *Acta Gastroenterol Latinoam*. 1997;27:67-73.
11. Trivedi MH, Lin EH, Katon WJ. Consensus recommendations for improving adherence, self-management, and outcomes in patients with depression. *CNS Spectr*. 2007;12:1-27.
12. Hedaya RJ. Pharmacokinetic factors in the clinical use of tryptophan. *J Clin Psychopharmacol*. 1984;4:347-348.
13. Frank E, Kupfer DJ, Perel JM, et al. Three-year outcomes for maintenance therapies in recurrent depression. *Arch Gen Psychiatry*. 1990;47:1093-1099.
14. Drabant EM, Hariri AR, Meyer-Lindenberg A, et al. Catechol O-methyltransferase val158met genotype and neural mechanisms related to affective arousal and regulation. *Arch Gen Psychiatry*. 2006;63:1396-1406.
15. Cussenot O, Azzouzi AR, Nicolaiew N, et al. Combination of polymorphisms from genes related to estrogen metabolism and risk of prostate cancers: the hidden face of estrogens. *J Clin Oncol*. 2007;25:3596-3602.
16. Ciolino H, MacDonald C, Memon O, Dankwah M, Yeh GC. Dehydroepiandrosterone inhibits the expression of carcinogen-activating enzymes in vivo. *Int J Cancer*. 2003;105:321-325.
17. Wentz MJ, Jamaluddin M, Garfield RE, Al-Hendy A. Regulation of catechol-O-methyltransferase expression in human myometrial cells. *Obstet Gynecol*. 2006;108:1439-1447.
18. Ellem SJ, Risbridger GP. Treating prostate cancer: a rationale for targeting local oestrogens. *Nat Rev Cancer*. 2007;7:621-627.

Appendix

Medical Symptoms Questionnaire

The Medical Symptoms Questionnaire can be used to determine the incidence of patient symptoms and their frequency, as well as to provide a quick measure of improvement when administered at regular intervals.

Name: _____   Date: _____

Rate each of the following symptoms based upon your typical health profile for:

❑ Past 30 days   ❑ Past 48 hours

Point Scale
0 - Never or almost never have the symptom
1 - Occasionally have it, effect is not severe
2 - Occasionally have it, effect is severe
3 - Frequently have it, effect is not severe
4 - Frequently have it, effect is severe

HEAD	_____ Headaches	Total _____
	_____ Faintness	
	_____ Dizziness	
	_____ Insomnia	

EYES	_____ Watery or itchy eyes	Total _____
	_____ Swollen, reddened or sticky eyelids	
	_____ Bags or dark circles under eyes	
	_____ Blurred or tunnel vision (does not include near- or far-sightedness)	

EARS	_____ Itchy ears	Total _____
	_____ Earaches, ear infections	
	_____ Drainage from ear	
	_____ Ringing in ears, hearing loss	

NOSE	_____ Stuffy nose	Total _____
	_____ Sinus problems	
	_____ Hay fever	
	_____ Sneezing attacks	
	_____ Excessive mucus formation	

MOUTH/THROAT	_____ Chronic coughing	Total _____
	_____ Gagging, frequent need to clear throat	
	_____ Sore throat, hoarseness, loss of voice	
	_____ Swollen or discolored tongue, gums, lips	
	_____ Canker sores	

SKIN	_____ Acne	Total _____
	_____ Hives, rashes, dry skin	
	_____ Hair loss	
	_____ Flushing, hot flashes	
	_____ Excessive sweating	

HEART	_____ Irregular or skipped heartbeat	Total _____
	_____ Rapid or pounding heartbeat	
	_____ Chest pain	

Medical Symptoms Questionnaire

LUNGS			
	_____	Chest congestion	Total _____
	_____	Asthma, bronchitis	
	_____	Shortness of breath	
	_____	Difficulty breathing	

DIGESTIVE TRACT			
	_____	Nausea, vomiting	Total _____
	_____	Diarrhea	
	_____	Constipation	
	_____	Bloated feeling	
	_____	Belching, passing gas	
	_____	Heartburn	
	_____	Intestinal/stomach pain	

JOINTS/MUSCLE			
	_____	Pain or aches in joints	Total _____
	_____	Arthritis	
	_____	Stiffness or limitation of movement	
	_____	Pain or aches in muscles	
	_____	Feeling of weakness or tiredness	

WEIGHT			
	_____	Binge eating/drinking	Total _____
	_____	Craving certain foods	
	_____	Excessive weight	
	_____	Compulsive eating	
	_____	Water retention	
	_____	Underweight	

ENERGY/ACTIVITY			
	_____	Fatigue, sluggishness	Total _____
	_____	Apathy, lethargy	
	_____	Hyperactivity	
	_____	Restlessness	

MIND			
	_____	Poor memory	Total _____
	_____	Confusion, poor comprehension	
	_____	Poor concentration	
	_____	Poor physical coordination	
	_____	Difficulty in making decisions	
	_____	Stuttering or stammering	
	_____	Slurred speech	
	_____	Learning disabilities	

EMOTIONS			
	_____	Mood swings	Total _____
	_____	Anxiety, fear, nervousness	
	_____	Anger, irritability, aggressiveness	
	_____	Depression	

OTHER			
	_____	Frequent illness	Total _____
	_____	Frequent or urgent urination	
	_____	Genital itch or discharge	

GRAND TOTAL _____

About the Authors

Robert J. Hedaya, MD, FAPA, has been teaching, practicing, and publishing in the field of psychiatry since 1980. He is board certified by the American Board of Adolescent Psychiatry, the American Board of Psychiatry and Neurology, and the American Society of Clinical Psychopharmacology. Dr. Hedaya is an active member of the Endocrine Society, a former consultant at the National Institute of Mental Health, a board member of the Suburban Maryland Psychiatric Society, and medical director of the New Hope Foundation. He is the founder of the National Center for Whole Psychiatry and a Clinical Professor of Psychiatry at Georgetown University Hospital in Washington, DC, where he has been selected as Outstanding Teacher of the Year on 3 occasions. Dr. Hedaya is the author of *Understanding Biological Psychiatry* (Norton, 1996) and *The Antidepressant Survival Guide* (Crown, 2000), and he lectures widely, including teaching at the annual International Symposium on Functional Medicine. He has made numerous media appearances (CNN, *60 Minutes*, *The Today Show*).

Dr. Hedaya has been practicing functional medicine as part of the whole psychiatry approach to psychiatric illness. This approach includes the allopathic psychiatric model and the functional medicine model as applied to psychiatry, as well as the depth psychological model (pioneered by Carl Jung). He believes that the healthcare model must continually be in flux, allowing for the introduction of new paradigms of healing. It is only with this approach that psychiatry can remain whole.

Sheila Quinn has held significant leadership positions in health-related nonprofit organizations over many years, including serving as Co-founder and Vice President at Bastyr University (1978–1990), Executive Director of the American Association of Naturopathic Physicians (1993–2000), and Senior Editor and Special Projects at The Institute for Functional Medicine (2000–2007). Her two passions are editing/writing and public policy advocacy. In pursuit of the latter, she helped to organize the Seattle Town Hall Meeting for the White House Commission on Complementary and Alternative Medicine Policy in October 2000, and she was on the Steering Committee for the 2001 National Policy Dialogue to Advance Integrated Health Care: Finding Common Ground (for which she coedited the final report). She is currently Board Chair for the Integrated Healthcare Policy Consortium. In her position at The Institute for Functional Medicine (IFM), she served as managing editor of the first-ever *Textbook of Functional Medicine* (for which she was also a contributing author); she was managing editor on the reissue of *Clinical Nutrition: A Functional Approach* (2nd ed.); she was a coauthor on "Healthy aging and the origins of illness: improving the expression of genetic potential" (*Integrative Medicine.* December 2003/January 2004;2:16-25); and she authored the self-study that gained IFM 6-year reaccreditation with commendation. In prior positions, she managed and edited journals, wrote numerous reports and self-studies, managed institutional finances and administrative services, and helped to advance the success of the many organizations to which she has devoted her time and energy. Through her 40-plus years of work both inside and outside the healthcare mainstream, she has become knowledgeable about both conventional and alternative medicine and health-related public policy issues, and she is committed to helping create a safe and effective integrated healthcare system. She is currently working as a freelance editor, writer, and public policy advocate and may be reached at sheila.quinn@comcast.net.